Workbook for Hartman's Complete Guide for the Phlebotomy Technician

by Hartman Publishing, Inc.

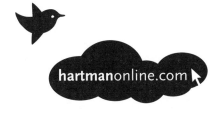

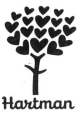

Credits

Managing Editor
Susan Alvare Hedman

Developmental Editor
Kristin Calderon

Cover Illustrator
Kirsten Browne

Production
Tracy Kopsachilis

Proofreaders
Juliann Barbato
Danielle Lescure
Zella Mansson

Copyright Information

© 2023 by Hartman Publishing, Inc.
1313 Iron Avenue SW
Albuquerque, New Mexico 87102
(505) 291-1274
web: hartmanonline.com
email: orders@hartmanonline.com
Twitter: @HartmanPub

All rights reserved. No part of this book may be reproduced, in any form or by any means, without permission in writing from the publisher.

ISBN 978-1-60425-161-6

PRINTED IN THE USA

Notice to Readers

Though the guidelines and procedures contained in this text are based on consultations with healthcare professionals, they should not be considered absolute recommendations. The instructor and readers should follow employer, local, state, and federal guidelines concerning healthcare practices. These guidelines change, and it is the reader's responsibility to be aware of these changes and of the policies and procedures of their healthcare facility.

The publisher, author, editors, and reviewers cannot accept any responsibility for errors or omissions or for any consequences from application of the information in this book and make no warranty, express or implied, with respect to the contents of the book. The publisher does not warrant or guarantee any of the products described herein or perform any analysis in connection with any of the product information contained herein.

Gender Usage

This workbook uses gender pronouns interchangeably to denote healthcare team members and patients.

Please do not copy our workbook. Report violations to legal@hartmanonline.com.

Table of Contents

Preface	v
1 Healthcare Settings and the Role of the Phlebotomy Technician	1
2 Legal and Ethical Issues	9
3 Communication and Patient Diversity	13
4 Infection Prevention and Control	21
5 Safety Measures for Care Team Members and Patients	27
6 Overview of the Human Body	31
7 The Circulatory System in Depth	37
8 Preparing for Specimen Collection	43
9 Collecting Blood Specimens by Venipuncture	53
10 Collecting Blood Specimens by Capillary (Dermal) Puncture	63
11 Nonblood Specimens	69
Procedure Checklists	75
Practice Exam	93

Preface

Welcome to the *Workbook for Hartman's Complete Guide for the Phlebotomy Technician*! This workbook is designed to help you review what you have learned from reading your textbook. For this reason, the workbook is organized around learning objectives, just like the textbook and your instructor's teaching material.

These learning objectives work as a built-in study guide. After completing the exercises for each learning objective in the workbook, ask yourself if you can *do* what that learning objective describes.

If you can, move on to the next learning objective. If you cannot, go back to the textbook, reread that learning objective, and try again.

We have provided procedure checklists close to the end of the workbook. There is also a practice test for the certification exam. The answers to the workbook exercises are in your instructor's teaching guide.

Happy learning!

Healthcare Settings and the Role of the Phlebotomy Technician

1. Discuss the healthcare system and describe changes in staffing trends

Multiple Choice
Circle the letter of the answer that best completes the statement or answers the question.

1. According to the Department of Labor, hiring of PBTs in the next several years
   (A) Will increase
   (B) Will go down
   (C) Will stay about the same
   (D) Will stop

2. Which of these kinds of healthcare workers are now doing routine patient care tasks that nurses may have done in the past?
   (A) Doctors and physician assistants
   (B) Occupational and speech therapists
   (C) Receptionists and coding specialists
   (D) Medical assistants and nursing assistants

3. This is one example of a *provider*:
   (A) A diagnostic laboratory
   (B) A home health agency
   (C) A hospital
   (D) A cardiac rehabilitation center

4. Who diagnoses illness and plans treatment?
   (A) A registered nurse
   (B) A medical assistant
   (C) An EKG technician
   (D) A doctor

5. Insurance companies, Medicare and Medicaid, and individual patients can all be _____ in the healthcare system.
   (A) Clients
   (B) Facilities
   (C) Payers
   (D) Providers

2. Describe common healthcare settings

Short Answer
For each of the items below, write O for outpatient or I for inpatient.

1. ____ In an emergency room, patients may be admitted to receive this type of care.

2. ____ A doctor's office provides this type of care.

3. ____ An urgent care center provides this type of care.

4. ____ This type of care is often needed for serious acute illnesses.

5. ____ Subacute care at a long-term care center is a form of this type of care.

6. ____ Standalone clinical laboratories where patients go for testing ordered by their doctors provide this type of care.

3. Discuss the organization and function of clinical laboratories

True or False
Mark each statement with either a T for true or an F for false.

1. ____ CLIA is a set of regulations that are meant to ensure the safety and accuracy of laboratory tests.

2. ____ All clinical laboratories are required to be accredited by either the Joint Commission or the College of American Pathologists.

3. ____ All clinical laboratories must meet CLIA standards.

4. _____ Medical technologists must have a doctoral degree, such as a PhD or MD.

5. _____ A clinical consultant at a diagnostic laboratory is responsible for day-to-day operations of the facility.

6. _____ Laboratories usually require that phlebotomy technicians be certified.

7. _____ Reference laboratories collect specimens but do not analyze them.

8. _____ Specimens commonly collected for analysis include blood, urine, stool, and sputum.

9. _____ Laboratories may also analyze specimens such as body tissues or cells.

Matching
For each of the numbered items, write the letter that best matches the term. Use each letter only once.

10. _____ Blood bank
11. _____ Chemistry
12. _____ Cytology
13. _____ Hematology
14. _____ Immunology
15. _____ Microbiology
16. _____ Pathology
17. _____ Stat
18. _____ Urinalysis

(A) Department where blood and other body fluids are tested for factors that affect the body's response to disease

(B) Department where tests are performed immediately so that urgently needed results are available quickly

(C) Department where blood is collected and prepared for transfusion

(D) Department where blood or other specimens may be cultured to analyze the microorganisms they contain

(E) Department where coagulation and the number and type of blood cells in a specimen may be analyzed

(F) Department that performs tests on urine

(G) Department where body tissues or other specimens are studied to determine the presence or progress of disease

(H) Department that would test blood for cholesterol, glucose, or hormone levels

(I) Department that studies cells for signs of disease

4. Discuss the healthcare team

Short Answer

1. List 2 types of certified healthcare workers other than phlebotomy technicians.

   _____
   _____
   _____

2. What do LVNs, LPNs, RNs, and physical therapists have in common in relation to credentials?

   _____
   _____
   _____

3. In addition to doctors, which healthcare professionals can generally examine patients, make diagnoses, and prescribe medications?

   _____
   _____
   _____

4. Which member of the healthcare team is also the reason the team exists?

   _____

5. Which 2 team members work together to ensure patients get the medications they need?

   _____
   _____

Name: _____

6. What does it mean for a phlebotomy technician to respect the facility's chain of command and stay within their scope of practice?

_____
_____
_____
_____
_____

5. Explain the phlebotomy technician's role

Multiple Choice

1. Which of the following describes a blood test that would be considered routine screening?
   (A) A long test to see how a pregnant woman processes glucose, given after results of a shorter test were abnormal
   (B) A blood culture to detect disease-causing microorganisms in the blood
   (C) A test to see if a blood thinner is working
   (D) A test to check cholesterol levels

2. A mobile phlebotomist's day may include
   (A) Staying at her regular station in a hospital laboratory, seeing 5 or 6 patients an hour
   (B) Going to different patients' rooms in the same hospital
   (C) Going to nursing homes, assisted living facilities, and patients' homes
   (D) Drawing blood in different examination rooms in a doctor's office

3. During venipuncture, phlebotomists collect blood specimens from blood
   (A) That is moving toward the patient's heart
   (B) That is moving away from the heart to the rest of the body
   (C) That is in the tiny blood vessels just beneath the skin
   (D) That is in the chambers of the heart

4. Which locations are commonly used when collecting specimens by dermal puncture?
   (A) The inside of the elbow or the back of the hand
   (B) The fingertip or the heel
   (C) The earlobe or the inside of the elbow
   (D) The back of the hand or the big toe

5. Who should answer any questions a patient has about why a doctor has ordered a test or what the results mean?
   (A) The phlebotomist who draws the patient's blood
   (B) The lab technician who performs the test
   (C) The clinical director of the laboratory
   (D) The provider who ordered the test

Short Answer

For each of the following tasks, write Y if a phlebotomy technician normally performs the task and N if a phlebotomy technician is not normally allowed to perform the task.

6. ____ Doing an arterial blood gas test

7. ____ Taking blood from a port or IV

8. ____ Answering a question such as, "How many tubes of blood do you need?"

9. ____ Being calm and reassuring while preparing a patient who is anxious about blood draws

10. ____ Making sure specimens are labeled correctly

11. ____ Explaining the process of drawing blood to the patient

12. ____ Inserting the needle to start an IV

13. ____ Giving the patient a routine vaccination by injection (e.g., a flu shot)

14. ____ Wearing gloves, disposing of needles correctly, and taking other measures to prevent the spread of infection

15. ____ Calling patients to give them test results

6. Explain policies and procedures

Fill in the Blank

1. A(n) _____ is a course of action that should be taken every time a certain situation occurs. A common one is that healthcare information must remain _____.

2. A(n) _____ is a method, or way, of doing something. For example, a facility will have one for reporting an incident such as a patient fainting during a blood draw.

3. Patient confidentiality is not only a facility rule; it is also the _____.

4. Phlebotomy technicians only collect specimens assigned on a(n) _____ form (which may be paper or electronic).

5. Healthcare workers should not do tasks that are not included in their job description. In other words, they must stay within their _____ _____.

7. Discuss the importance of quality assurance and quality improvement in healthcare organizations

Short Answer

1. What is the difference between *quality assurance* and *quality improvement*?

   _____
   _____
   _____
   _____

2. What is the name for processes put into place to document that standards are being met at a facility?

   _____
   _____

3. What is one way for a facility to prove that it meets the federal government's quality standards?

   _____
   _____
   _____

4. Are CLIA and CLSI the same thing? Explain your answer.

   _____
   _____
   _____
   _____
   _____
   _____

5. What are the 3 aims of the National Quality Strategy?

   _____
   _____
   _____

6. What are 3 things phlebotomy technicians can do to help meet continuous quality improvement goals at their facilities?

   _____
   _____
   _____
   _____
   _____

8. Describe certification, recertification, and continuing education for the phlebotomy technician

Multiple Choice

1. Which of the following is true of certification for phlebotomy technicians?
   (A) It is required by the federal government.
   (B) It is required by all state governments.
   (C) It is required by some states and many facilities.
   (D) It is only necessary if a phlebotomy technician plans to eventually become a nurse or doctor.

Name: _____

2. Before a phlebotomist may be certified, most certification agencies require
   (A) Proof of clinical experience, including venipuncture and capillary puncture
   (B) Proof of clinical experience, including venipuncture, capillary puncture, and arterial puncture
   (C) An interview and oral examination
   (D) Completion of an essay about the circulatory system

3. Which of these factors is most important for a student to consider when choosing a certification agency?
   (A) Whether their state requires certification through a particular agency
   (B) Whether the certification agency provides a pin or other symbol of program completion
   (C) How long the test will be
   (D) Whether there are online study materials available

4. After receiving certification in phlebotomy, a phlebotomy technician
   (A) Will never have to take another class or test
   (B) Will never have to renew certification
   (C) Can continue to be certified whether or not she works as a phlebotomist
   (D) Must work as a phlebotomist and participate in continuing education to renew certification

5. Who is responsible for making sure a PBT meets deadlines and fulfills requirements for recertification?
   (A) The PBT's instructor
   (B) The PBT
   (C) The PBT's employer
   (D) The certification agency

6. Before being certified as a phlebotomy technician, a student must usually
   (A) Get a bachelor's degree
   (B) Get an associate degree
   (C) Get a high school diploma (or GED)
   (D) Serve in the military

9. Explain professionalism and list examples of professional behavior

Short Answer

1. What is the difference between *personal* and *professional*?
   _____
   _____
   _____
   _____

2. List 3 reasons why it is important for phlebotomy technicians to demonstrate professionalism.
   _____
   _____
   _____
   _____
   _____

3. Choose one of the qualities listed on pp. 13–14 of the textbook and describe a situation in which that quality may be shown. For example, for *patient* the situation could be explaining the procedure carefully and taking the necessary time when drawing blood from a child who is fearful.
   _____
   _____
   _____
   _____
   _____
   _____

For each of the items below, write P for examples of professional behavior with a patient and E for examples of professional behavior with an employer.

4. ____ Communicating when unable to get to work on time

5. ____ Not discussing possibly controversial topics such as politics or religion

6. _____ Explaining procedures before beginning
7. _____ Completing tasks efficiently
8. _____ Participating in educational programs
9. _____ Not discussing information that is beyond a phlebotomy technician's scope of practice
10. _____ Being a positive role model for the facility
11. _____ Listening to concerns and taking them seriously
12. _____ Documenting and reporting carefully and correctly
13. _____ Reporting anything that keeps a PBT from completing duties
14. _____ Following the chain of command
15. _____ Adjusting communication based on age or condition

10. Describe proper personal grooming habits

Fill in the Blank

1. A phlebotomy technician's grooming habits affect how _____ patients feel about the care given.
2. Perfume, cologne, aftershave, and scented body creams or lotions _____ _____ be used.
3. The main exception to a *no large jewelry* rule is a simple _____.
4. Long hair should be kept in a(n) _____ or a(n) _____.
5. PBTs should wear comfortable, clean, high-quality, _____ shoes.
6. Artificial nails and nail wraps should not be worn because they harbor _____. Nails should be kept _____, smooth, and clean.
7. Facial hair should be _____, _____, and _____.
8. These oral hygiene practices are important: _____ teeth and using _____ when necessary.
9. PBTs must wear a(n) _____ _____ as required by their facility. This allows patients to know who is caring for them.
10. Uniforms should be clean and _____.

11. Demonstrate how to manage time and assignments

True or False

1. _____ Each patient a PBT sees may need different tests and require individual attention.
2. _____ When patients have orders for multiple tests, specimen tubes may be filled in any order.
3. _____ Errors are more likely when a PBT does not take time to organize and check supplies before a blood draw.
4. _____ PBTs should always be able to complete their work without asking for help.

12. List appropriate ways to deal with stress

Multiple Choice

1. Which of the following is an example of a positive situation that is likely to cause stress?
   (A) Having a free weekend with no homework or housework to do
   (B) Receiving a gift card as a birthday present
   (C) Graduating from a career training program
   (D) Losing a job

Name: _____

2. A type of patient who may create stress during a phlebotomy technician's day is one who
   (A) Is extremely anxious about a possible diagnosis and is having a hard time staying still
   (B) Has had blood drawn many times and is not fearful
   (C) Does not like blood draws but is eager to have the draw over with
   (D) Makes small talk and looks away to manage mild fear of the procedure

3. What should a person identify before making a plan to manage stress?
   (A) Sources of stress for the people around them
   (B) Gyms and community centers in their neighborhood
   (C) Recipes for their favorite comfort meals
   (D) Sources and effects of stress in their life

4. What may be said about alcohol and stress management?
   (A) Alcohol should not be consumed at all.
   (B) Alcohol should be consumed only in moderation.
   (C) Alcohol should be consumed in large quantities.
   (D) Alcohol should only be consumed in social situations.

5. Which of the following may be a sign of stress not being managed well?
   (A) Getting 8–9 hours of sleep each night
   (B) Meeting friends for a beer after work on a Friday
   (C) Having a short temper with patients and coworkers
   (D) Feeling better after taking a long walk every day

6. Phlebotomy technicians should not talk to _____ about personal or job-related stress.
   (A) Coworkers
   (B) Supervisors
   (C) A therapist
   (D) Patients

Short Answer

7. List 4 sources of stress in your life. Try to think of at least 1 source of stress that is something positive. For each item, note whether it is something you can change.

   _____
   _____
   _____
   _____
   _____
   _____

8. What do you find helpful to manage stress? Do different stressors require different management techniques?

   _____
   _____
   _____
   _____
   _____
   _____

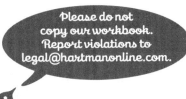

2

Legal and Ethical Issues

1. Define the terms *law* and *ethics* and list examples of legal and ethical behavior

Short Answer

For each of the following examples, decide whether the issue is a legal or an ethical issue. Write L for legal or E for ethical.

1. ____ When Maria is at home with her husband she makes fun of the way one of the patients she sees speaks English.

2. ____ Dennis takes a book from a patient's purse while she is using the bathroom and gives it to a friend.

3. ____ Imani is 10 minutes late coming in for work on Monday. Her supervisor does not notice and Imani does not tell her.

4. ____ Rachel is excited to see that a well-known musician is a patient at the facility where she works. She opens his record and takes a photo to show her friends.

Read the scenarios below and then answer the questions that follow.

Sarah, a PBT at a children's hospital, is out shopping with her friends. One of them asks her if she likes her job, and she responds enthusiastically. She then tells them about Jonah, a young patient with leukemia, and how inspired she is by his courage. She tells them about all the tests and treatments Jonah has to go through.

5. Did Sarah behave in a legal and ethical manner? Why or why not?

_____

_____

_____

_____

The day Jonah is discharged from the hospital where Sarah works, his mother takes Sarah aside. She says that she really appreciates how kind Sarah has been during such a difficult time for their family. She tells her that she is one of Jonah's favorites at the hospital, even though she had to draw blood, which scared him. She gives her a wrapped present and says it is to show their gratitude. Sarah initially refuses, but after the mother insists, she takes it from her, thanking her.

6. Did Sarah behave in a legal and ethical manner? Why or why not?

_____

_____

_____

_____

2. Explain HIPAA and discuss ways to protect patients' privacy

Multiple Choice

1. What is included under protected health information (PHI)?
   (A) Patient's favorite food
   (B) Patient's favorite color
   (C) Patient's social security number
   (D) Patient's library card number

Legal and Ethical Issues

2. What is one purpose of the Health Insurance Portability and Accountability Act (HIPAA)?
   (A) To monitor quality of care in medical facilities
   (B) To protect and secure the privacy of health information
   (C) To reduce incidents of patient abuse
   (D) To provide health insurance for uninsured elderly people

3. What is the correct response by a phlebotomy technician if someone who is not directly involved with a patient's care asks for a patient's PHI?
   (A) Give them the information
   (B) Ask the patient if they may have the information
   (C) Ask them to ask someone else
   (D) Tell them that the information is confidential and cannot be shared

4. Which of the following is one way to keep private health information confidential?
   (A) Making comments about patients on Twitter
   (B) Discussing patients' possible diagnoses with a coworker in a restaurant
   (C) Using private rooms for discussing patient information
   (D) Only discussing patients' conditions with trusted family members

5. The abbreviation for a law that was enacted as a part of the American Recovery and Reinvestment Act of 2009 to expand the protection and security of consumers' electronic health records (EHR) is
   (A) HISEAL
   (B) HITECH
   (C) HIHELP
   (D) HIQUIET

6. Penalties for violating HIPAA may include
   (A) A verbal warning
   (B) Prison sentences up to 10 months
   (C) Fines up to $100
   (D) Fines from $100 to $1.5 million and prison sentences up to 10 years

3. Explain the Clinical Laboratory Improvement Amendments (CLIA) and laboratory certification

Fill in the Blank

1. The goal of CLIA is to improve _____ _____ by ensuring that laboratory tests are performed by _____ personnel and follow _____, effective procedures.

2. Tests that are simple, easy to perform, and have little risk of _____ are known as CLIA _____ _____.

3. Phlebotomy technicians may perform some of these tests. Many of them are _____ tests, meaning they are done near or in the presence of the patient.

4. The highest level of CLIA certification is the _____ _____ _____ for facilities performing moderate- to high-_____ tests.

5. The American Society for Clinical Laboratory Science's goals for quality laboratory testing include the following:
   - Perform the _____ test.
   - Perform the test on the right _____.
   - Perform the test at the right _____.
   - Produce _____ test results.
   - Achieve the best _____.
   - Perform the test in the most _____ manner.

6. Phlebotomy technicians contribute to meeting quality standards by _____ their scope of practice, not performing tasks for which they are not _____, and following their facility's _____ and _____ at all times.

Name: _____

4. Discuss common legal considerations in health care, including negligence, abuse, and consent

Matching
Use each letter only once.

1. _____ Tort
2. _____ Civil law
3. _____ Criminal law
4. _____ Consent
5. _____ Informed consent
6. _____ Express consent
7. _____ Implied consent
8. _____ Negligence
9. _____ Abuse
10. _____ Assault
11. _____ Battery

(A) Consent that is actively, consciously given

(B) Actions, or the failure to act, that result in injury

(C) Violation of civil law

(D) Consent that is assumed based on what a "reasonable person" would agree to in order to protect their life and well-being; used when treating a person who is unconscious or a minor whose guardian is not present

(E) Deals with offenses considered to harm all of society

(F) Acknowledgement that a patient understands the treatment they will receive and agrees to receive it

(G) The intentional touching of a person without permission

(H) Purposeful mistreatment that causes physical, mental, or emotional pain or injury to someone

(I) Deals with disputes between individuals

(J) The use of words or actions to cause another person to feel fearful of being harmed

(K) In health care, a general term for a patient's agreement to being treated

Multiple Choice

12. When providing care to a minor, a phlebotomy technician should understand that
    (A) Minors over the age of 12 can consent to medical care for themselves
    (B) Parents or guardians consent on behalf of minors
    (C) Consent is not required when providing medical care for minors
    (D) Any adult family member may consent on behalf of minors

13. Which of the following adults is most likely to have a legal representative who provides consent?
    (A) A patient with an intellectual disability who lives independently and works at a supermarket
    (B) A patient who takes medication to treat a mental health disorder
    (C) A patient who just turned 18
    (D) A patient who is in the late stages of Alzheimer's disease and cannot always state his own name

5. Explain the American Hospital Association's Patient Care Partnership and discuss why patient rights are important

Short Answer
Read the scenarios below and then answer the questions that follow.

Theresa is a phlebotomy technician at a hospital. She is sent to the room of Ms. Land, an elderly woman in the hospital for pneumonia, to draw blood for tests ordered by the doctor. Ms. Land says she is tired of being poked and examined and she will not have her blood drawn. Theresa tells her she is being very naughty and that she may have to call a strong friend to help her draw Ms. Land's blood.

1. Which of Ms. Land's rights are being violated? What could Theresa do instead?

_____
_____
_____
_____
_____

Ms. Land refuses to have her blood drawn. Theresa had already prepared the equipment for the blood draw. She takes the open, assembled needle and tube holder to the room of Mr. Diewald, the next patient she is assigned to draw.

2. Do you think this may be a violation of Mr. Diewald's rights? In what way?

_____
_____
_____
_____
_____

Malik is a new phlebotomist at a diagnostic laboratory. When he calls his first patient, he enters the waiting room and says loudly, "Stephen Higley, for a PT/INR?"

3. Is this a violation of Mr. Higley's rights? If so, what should Malik do differently?

_____
_____
_____
_____
_____
_____

For each of the following situations, describe how a PBT could respond in a way that protects the patient's rights.

4. A hospital patient has orders for a blood culture. Blood culture samples are collected in special bottles. The patient has never seen this before and has questions about why the test was ordered and how it works.

_____
_____
_____
_____
_____
_____
_____

5. A patient's medical record lists the name Kathryn (Kate) Baker. When the PBT says, "Hi, Kate, how are you today?" the patient says he is fine, but that he prefers to be called Kade and uses he/him pronouns.

_____
_____
_____
_____
_____
_____

6. A patient says her blood is often hard to draw and that she'd prefer the PBT to use her left arm. She says phlebotomists have had better luck with her left arm in the past. The PBT finds it easier to draw from patients' right arms.

_____
_____
_____
_____
_____
_____
_____

Please do not copy our workbook. Report violations to legal@hartmanonline.com.

3

Communication and Patient Diversity

1. Define *communication* and understand the importance of both verbal and nonverbal communication

Short Answer

1. List the 3 basic steps of communication.

   _____
   _____
   _____

2. Why is feedback an important part of communication?

   _____
   _____
   _____
   _____

3. With whom must phlebotomy technicians be able to communicate?

   _____
   _____
   _____
   _____

Multiple Choice

4. Which 3 things are needed for communication to take place?
   (A) Signs, symbols, and drawings
   (B) Sender, receiver, and feedback
   (C) Provider, patients, and family members
   (D) Loud voice, ability to speak, and patient's chart

5. The 3-step process of communication
   (A) Happens only once
   (B) Happens over and over
   (C) Only happens in formal meetings
   (D) Happens in a different order every time

6. Which of the following is an example of nonverbal communication?
   (A) Asking for a glass of water
   (B) Pointing to a glass of water
   (C) Screaming for a glass of water
   (D) Saying "I do not like water."

7. Verbal communication includes
   (A) Facial expressions
   (B) Nodding one's head
   (C) Speaking
   (D) Shrugging one's shoulders

8. Types of nonverbal communication include
   (A) Speaking
   (B) Facial expressions
   (C) Yelling
   (D) Oral reports

9. Which of the following is an example of a confusing or conflicting message (saying one thing and meaning another)?
   (A) Mr. Carter smiles and says he is happy to have his blood drawn because he is sure his cholesterol numbers are down.
   (B) Mrs. Sanchez looks like she is in pain as a PBT feels for a vein. When the PBT asks her about it, Mrs. Sanchez says she had a bruise on that arm that still hurts.
   (C) Ms. Jones agrees with the PBT when she says it is a nice day, but she looks upset.
   (D) Mr. Lee will not look up from the floor. He says he is a little worried about his blood test.

10. In the previous question, what is the most likely reason for the confusing or conflicting message?
    (A) The patient is a person who does not tell the truth.
    (B) The person means what they said and just has a grumpy manner.
    (C) The person dislikes the phlebotomy technician.
    (D) The person is anxious about the blood draw or about their health.

Short Answer
State whether each behavior below sends a positive message or a negative message to the receiver. Write P for positive and N for negative.

11. _____ Using an impatient tone
12. _____ Smiling
13. _____ Leaning forward in a chair
14. _____ Glancing repeatedly at a watch
15. _____ Sitting up straight
16. _____ Slouching
17. _____ Crossing arms in front of the body
18. _____ Listening carefully
19. _____ Nodding the head
20. _____ Rolling eyes

2. Identify barriers to communication and understand different communication styles and preferences

Crossword
Across

3. Type of terminology that may not be understood by patients or their families
5. Types of questions that should be asked because they elicit more than a "yes" or "no" answer
7. Phrases used over and over again that do not really mean anything

Down

1. Type of language, along with gestures and facial expressions, that is part of nonverbal communication
2. Being this way and taking time to listen when patients are difficult to understand helps promote better communication.
4. PBTs cannot offer opinions or give this because it is not within their scope of practice.
6. PBTs should not ask this when patients make statements because it often makes people feel defensive.
8. Along with profanity, these types of words and expressions should not be used by PBTs.

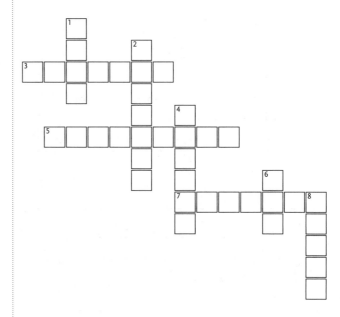

Short Answer

9. Choose one of the steps to ensure accurate communication listed on pp. 33–34 of the textbook. Describe a time when you have used one of these steps to improve communication.

_____
_____
_____
_____
_____

10. Choose another of the steps to ensure accurate communication. Describe a scenario (other than those listed in the textbook) when you think it may be helpful in your work as a phlebotomy technician.

_____

_____

_____

_____

3. Understand common medical terminology and abbreviations

Multiple Choice

1. With whom should a PBT use medical terminology?
   (A) With patients
   (B) With patients' family members
   (C) With other care team members
   (D) With the facility's business manager

2. What is one advantage of a PBT using medical terms when appropriate?
   (A) It is like a secret language that makes it more difficult for patients to understand.
   (B) It makes the best use of the PBT's training.
   (C) It makes communication more specific and accurate.
   (D) It shows others that the PBT is intelligent.

Fill in the Blank

3. A(n) _____ is the part of a word that contains its basic meaning or definition.

4. The _____ is the word part that precedes (comes before) the root to help form a new word.

5. The _____ is the word part added to the end of a root that helps form a new word.

Short Answer

6. *Erythro-* means red and *-cyte* means cell. What do you think an erythrocyte is?

_____

7. *Hemat(o)* means blood and *-oma* means swelling or mass. What do you think a hematoma is?

_____

4. Explain documentation and describe related terms and forms

Multiple Choice

1. If a mistake is made when documenting on paper, the PBT should
   (A) Erase what she has written and enter the correct information
   (B) Draw a line through the error and initial and date it
   (C) Use white correction fluid to cover the error and then initial and date the white area
   (D) Staple a new sheet to the front of the medical chart that has the correct information

2. When is it appropriate for a PBT to document a procedure before it has been done?
   (A) When a patient requests it
   (B) Never
   (C) When there are lots of patients waiting
   (D) When more than 5 tubes will be drawn

3. What color of ink is the best choice for documenting by hand?
   (A) Red
   (B) Black
   (C) Purple
   (D) Green

4. Which statement is an example of a fact?
   (A) Ms. Lopez was not happy about getting her blood drawn.
   (B) Ms. Lopez seemed dehydrated.
   (C) Ms. Lopez has bad veins.
   (D) PBT was not able to complete venipuncture and called the nurse after 2 failed attempts.

5. Which of the following is the correct way to express 2:00 p.m. using the 24-hour clock?
   (A) 0200
   (B) 2.00
   (C) 1400
   (D) 14.5

6. A blood draw that is documented as having happened at 1650 hours was done at
   (A) 4:50 p.m.
   (B) 4:30 p.m.
   (C) 6:50 a.m.
   (D) 6:50 p.m.

7. When documenting on a computer or tablet, the PBT should know that
   (A) Confidentiality is not a concern because computers are more secure than paper charts
   (B) Confidentiality is only a concern if a facility has been targeted by hackers in the past
   (C) HIPAA guidelines do not apply to computer documentation
   (D) HIPAA guidelines apply to computer documentation and confidentiality must be protected

True or False

8. _____ A phlebotomy technician can choose whether or not to report an incident.

9. _____ Collecting a specimen from the wrong patient would be considered an incident.

10. _____ An incident report includes a description of the incident itself but does not document the response to the incident.

11. _____ Incident reports can help prevent future incidents.

12. _____ The information in an incident report should not be included in a patient's medical record.

5. List guidelines for communicating with different populations

Multiple Choice

Hearing Impairment

1. To best communicate with a patient who has a hearing impairment, the phlebotomy technician should
   (A) Use short sentences and simple words
   (B) Shout
   (C) Approach the patient from behind
   (D) Raise the pitch of her voice

2. If a patient is difficult to understand, the PBT should
   (A) Pretend to understand the patient so as not to hurt his feelings
   (B) Mouth the words in an exaggerated way so that the patient will mimic that behavior next time
   (C) Ask the patient to repeat what he said, and then tell the patient what the PBT thinks she heard
   (D) Ask the patient to speak up

3. Which of the following settings would be best for communicating with a patient with hearing impairment?
   (A) A busy waiting room
   (B) A quiet exam room
   (C) An area where other team members are often coming and going
   (D) The employee break room

Vision Impairment

4. Which of the following is true of patients with vision impairment?
   (A) They will all be elderly.
   (B) They will be unable to see anything at all.
   (C) They may wear contact lenses or eyeglasses.
   (D) They do not need to be told what is happening around them.

Name: _____

5. Where should a PBT stand while talking to a patient with a vision impairment?
   (A) To the patient's side
   (B) Behind the patient
   (C) In front of the patient, facing him
   (D) In front of the patient, looking down at the requisition

6. When performing a blood draw on a patient who has a vision impairment, the phlebotomy technician should
   (A) Touch the patient, then identify herself
   (B) Be quiet so as not to startle the patient
   (C) Wait until she is very close to the patient, then touch the patient on the arm
   (D) Identify herself immediately, before touching the patient

7. Which of the following would be appropriate for a PBT to say when drawing blood from a patient with vision impairment?
   (A) "You're going to feel me touching your arm now to find a vein."
   (B) "Stay still and I'll let you know when this is over."
   (C) "I guess I don't have to tell you to look away if you don't like needles!"
   (D) "As you can see, we don't have many tubes to fill. This will be quick."

Fill in the Blank

Cognitive Impairment

8. Always approach from the front, and do not _____ _____ _____.

9. Always _____ _____ and use the patient's name. Continue to _____ _____ _____ _____ as you provide care.

10. Speak slowly, using a lower _____ _____ _____ than normal. This is _____ and easier to understand.

11. Repeat yourself, using the same _____ _____ _____, as often as necessary.

12. Use signs, pictures, gestures, or _____ _____ to help communicate as needed.

13. Ask any family member or caregiver accompanying the patient for _____ about communication with the patient, as appropriate.

True or False

Pediatric Patients

14. ___ It is important to be reassuring and to take time to help young patients manage their anxiety.

15. ___ Young children should not be allowed to sit in a parent or caregiver's lap during a blood draw.

16. ___ It is not necessary for a phlebotomy technician to introduce himself to a pediatric patient.

17. ___ It can help for the phlebotomy technician to lower herself physically to the child's eye level.

18. ___ A PBT should always speak to the parent or caregiver rather than directly to the child.

19. ___ It is helpful to tell the child there will be a prize if they are brave and do not cry.

20. ___ One helpful technique is to say you will not draw blood after all and then put the needle in when the child is not looking.

21. ___ It is never acceptable to shame or threaten a child.

Multiple Choice

Geriatric Patients

22. Which of the following is true of geriatric patients?
    (A) They all have some kind of impairment.
    (B) They are not likely to remember what happens during a medical appointment.
    (C) They will all have similar conditions and attitudes.
    (D) They are all individuals and it is important not to make assumptions about them.

23. If a patient comes to an appointment with an adult child or other caregiver, how should the PBT behave with that person?
    (A) The PBT should address all communication to the child/caregiver.
    (B) The PBT should not address the child/caregiver at all.
    (C) The PBT should answer the child's/caregiver's questions but communicate directly with the patient.
    (D) The PBT should request that the child/caregiver stay in the waiting room.

24. Which of the following is an appropriate way to address Mr. Trujillo, an elderly patient?
    (A) Gramps
    (B) Honey
    (C) Sweetie
    (D) Mr. Trujillo

Short Answer

Patients with Developmental Disabilities
State whether each behavior below is an appropriate way to communicate with patients with developmental disabilities. Write A for appropriate and N for not appropriate.

25. _____ Not describing procedures so as not to cause the patient concern

26. _____ Remaining calm and patient

27. _____ Treating adult patients with intellectual disabilities as if they were children

28. _____ Assuming the patient will not have any questions

29. _____ Telling a patient with autism spectrum disorder to look at you when she speaks

30. _____ Watching for nonverbal cues that the patient is anxious or confused

True or False

Patients Who Speak Limited or No English

31. _____ According to the US Census Bureau, less than 10% of adults in the United States speak a language other than English in their homes.

32. _____ Patients have a right to receive information about their medical care in a language they understand.

33. _____ Patients who do not understand what a PBT is saying will always say that they do not understand.

34. _____ Family members or friends of the patient can be relied on for medical translation.

35. _____ It is helpful for a PBT to learn a few words or phrases of languages commonly spoken in the community where they work.

36. _____ Medical offices and facilities should have interpretation services available.

Short Answer

Patients Who Are Combative, Angry, or Inappropriate

37. List 4 possible causes of combative or inappropriate behavior in a patient.

_____

_____

_____

_____

38. How should a phlebotomy technician respond if a patient makes an inappropriate or sexual comment?

_____

_____

_____

_____

39. What should a PBT do if a patient attempts to physically strike them?

_____

_____

_____

Name: _____

40. In what situation should a PBT report inappropriate behavior to a supervisor?

_____
_____
_____
_____

Name: _____

4

Infection Prevention and Control

1. Define *infection prevention* and discuss types of infections

Matching
Use each letter only once.

1. ____ Healthcare-associated infection
2. ____ Infection
3. ____ Infection prevention
4. ____ Localized infection
5. ____ Microorganism/microbe
6. ____ Pathogen
7. ____ Systemic infection
8. ____ *Clostridioides difficile* (*C. diff*)

(A) Set of methods practiced in healthcare facilities to prevent and control the spread of disease

(B) A harmful microorganism

(C) An infection acquired in a healthcare setting during the delivery of medical care

(D) A small living thing that is only visible under a microscope

(E) An infection that travels through the bloodstream and is spread throughout the body

(F) Occurs when pathogens invade and multiply within the body

(G) An infection that is limited to a specific location in the body

(H) A spore-forming pathogen that can cause diarrhea and nausea and is a common healthcare-associated infection

2. Describe the chain of infection

Multiple Choice

1. The following are necessary links in the chain of infection. Which link is broken by wearing gloves, thus preventing the spread of disease?
   (A) Reservoir (place where the pathogen lives and grows)
   (B) Mode of transmission (a way for the disease to spread)
   (C) Susceptible host (person who is likely to get the disease)
   (D) Portal of exit (body opening that allows pathogens to leave)

2. The following are necessary links in the chain of infection. By getting a vaccination for hepatitis B, which link will a person affect to prevent him from getting this disease?
   (A) Reservoir (place where the pathogen lives and grows)
   (B) Mode of transmission (a way for the disease to spread)
   (C) Susceptible host (person who is likely to get the disease)
   (D) Portal of exit (body opening that allows pathogens to leave)

3. Handwashing with regular soap and water is one form of
   (A) Medical asepsis
   (B) Personal protective equipment
   (C) Surgical asepsis
   (D) Sterile technique

4. In what type of environment do microorganisms grow best?
   (A) In a warm, moist place
   (B) In a bright place
   (C) In a cool, dry place
   (D) In a frozen place

3. Explain Standard Precautions

True or False

1. ____ Following Standard Precautions means treating blood and other body fluids, nonintact skin, and mucous membranes as if they were infected.

2. ____ Under Standard Precautions, body fluids do not include saliva.

3. ____ A phlebotomy technician can usually tell if someone has an infectious illness just by looking at him.

4. ____ A phlebotomy technician should wash her hands before donning (putting on) gloves.

5. ____ A phlebotomy technician should carefully recap used syringes before putting them in a biohazard container.

6. ____ Drawing blood is one task that requires a PBT to wear gloves.

7. ____ A mask and goggles are never worn during phlebotomy procedures.

8. ____ Biomedical/biohazard waste that is not sharp should be discarded in a regular trash bag.

Multiple Choice

9. Standard Precautions should be practiced
   (A) Only on patients who look like they have a bloodborne disease
   (B) On every single patient a phlebotomy technician encounters
   (C) Only on patients who request that the phlebotomy technician follow them
   (D) Only on patients who have tuberculosis

10. Standard Precautions include the following:
    (A) Washing hands after taking off gloves but not before putting on gloves
    (B) Wearing gloves if there is a possibility of coming into contact with blood or other body fluids, mucous membranes, or broken skin
    (C) Touching body fluids with bare hands
    (D) Disposing of sharps in plastic bags marked *biohazard*

11. Which of the following is true of both Standard Precautions and Transmission-Based Precautions?
    (A) They are different names for the same thing.
    (B) They stop an infected person from giving off pathogens.
    (C) They can prevent pathogens from an infected patient from infecting others.
    (D) They vary by state and facility.

12. How should sharps be discarded?
    (A) Sharps should be placed in blue recycling containers.
    (B) Sharps should be placed in trash containers in parts of the facility that are not used often.
    (C) Sharps should be placed inside used gloves and then in hazardous waste bags.
    (D) Sharps should be placed in puncture-resistant biohazard containers.

13. The Occupational Safety and Health Administration (OSHA) is a federal government agency that protects workers from
    (A) Unfair employment practices
    (B) Sexual harassment
    (C) Workplace violence
    (D) Hazards on the job

4. Explain hand hygiene and identify when to wash hands

Short Answer

1. What is the most common way for healthcare-associated infections to spread?

_____

_____

Name: _____

2. Give at least one reason why hand sanitizer is not a substitute for frequent, proper handwashing.

   _____
   _____

3. List 4 things a PBT might wear that could harbor bacteria.

   _____
   _____
   _____
   _____

4. PBT Devon arrives at work at 7:30 a.m. She goes to the employee break room and gets a cup of coffee and a muffin. She checks her station to restock supplies. She checks her scheduled appointments for the day and, knowing there will also be walk-ins, sees that she will be very busy. It is 7:50 and appointments begin at 8:00, so she visits the restroom. At 8:00 she calls her first patient. Her second patient is already waiting. By the time Devon draws blood for the second patient, how many times will she have washed her hands, at a minimum? List each time.

   _____
   _____
   _____
   _____
   _____

5. Discuss the use of personal protective equipment (PPE)

Short Answer
Place a check mark (✓) next to the tasks that require a phlebotomy technician to wear gloves.

1. _____ Contact with body fluids
2. _____ When the PBT may touch blood
3. _____ Greeting and identifying a patient
4. _____ Answering the telephone
5. _____ Taking a requisition from the patient and reading it
6. _____ Delivering a sealed bag of blood collection tubes to the laboratory for analysis
7. _____ Collecting a sputum specimen (a specimen of mucus coughed up by the patient)
8. _____ Drawing blood
9. _____ Opening a new box of collection tubes

Multiple Choice

10. What type of PPE may be needed when caring for a patient with a respiratory illness?
    (A) Eyeglasses and mask
    (B) Mask and foot covering
    (C) Eyeglasses and gloves
    (D) Mask and goggles

11. What type of PPE is used most often by healthcare workers?
    (A) Gloves
    (B) Mask
    (C) Face shield
    (D) Goggles

12. How many times can a gown be worn before it needs to be discarded?
    (A) 1 time
    (B) 2 times
    (C) 3 times
    (D) 4 times

13. If blood or body fluids may be splashed or sprayed into the eye area, proper protection for the eyes is
    (A) Eyeglasses
    (B) Mask
    (C) Sunglasses
    (D) Goggles

Short Answer

14. What is the correct order for donning (putting on) PPE (gloves, mask, gown, goggles)?

    _____
    _____

15. What is the correct order for doffing (removing) PPE (gloves, mask, gown, goggles)?

_____

_____

16. Which type of PPE is removed *after* exiting a patient's room?

_____

6. Explain Transmission-Based Precautions

Short Answer

List the type of precaution being described in each phrase below. Use an A for Airborne Precautions, a C for Contact Precautions, and a D for Droplet Precautions. Each letter may be used more than once.

1. ____ Transmission can occur when touching a contaminated area on the patient's body.

2. ____ Used when there is a risk of spreading an infection by direct contact with a person or object

3. ____ Used to guard against tuberculosis

4. ____ Covering the nose and mouth with a tissue when a person sneezes or coughs and washing hands immediately after sneezing are parts of these precautions.

5. ____ Help prevent the spread of *Clostridioides difficile* (*C. diff*) and conjunctivitis

6. ____ Used when the microorganisms are spread by droplets in the air that travel only short distances (normally not more than 6 feet)

7. ____ Microorganisms can be spread by coughing, sneezing, talking, laughing, or suctioning.

8. ____ Help prevent the spread of illnesses transmitted by pathogens that stay floating in the air for some time after being expelled

9. ____ Help protect against transmission of influenza

10. ____ May require the use of a special mask, such as an N95 or HEPA mask

Multiple Choice

11. Transmission-Based Precautions are used
    (A) With every patient a phlebotomy technician encounters
    (B) In addition to Standard Precautions
    (C) Instead of Standard Precautions
    (D) When a PBT decides that they are appropriate for particular patients

12. Which of the following is true of equipment that is not disposable and is used in caring for multiple patients?
    (A) It can never be used on patients with known infectious illnesses.
    (B) It can only be used by physicians and other licensed medical professionals.
    (C) It must be disinfected on a daily basis.
    (D) It must be disinfected after each use.

13. Which of the following is true of wearing PPE while caring for patients in isolation?
    (A) Phlebotomy technicians will have to decide for themselves which PPE they must wear while caring for patients in isolation.
    (B) Phlebotomy technicians should remove most PPE before exiting an isolation room.
    (C) Phlebotomy technicians will always wear the same PPE while caring for all patients in isolation.
    (D) Phlebotomy technicians should remove all PPE after exiting an isolation room.

7. Define *bloodborne pathogens* and describe two major bloodborne diseases

Fill in the Blank

1. Bloodborne diseases cannot be spread by _____ _____.

2. Bloodborne pathogens are _____ found in human blood that can cause _____ and _____ in humans.

Name: _____

3. In health care, contact with infected _____ or _____ _____ is the most common way to be infected with a bloodborne disease.

4. The final stage of HIV infection is _____. At this stage, people lose all ability to _____ _____ and can die from illnesses that a healthy _____ _____ could handle.

5. Hepatitis is inflammation of the _____ caused by certain _____ and other factors, such as alcohol abuse, some medications, and trauma.

6. Employers must offer phlebotomy technicians a free vaccine to protect them from _____.

7. HBV is a serious threat to healthcare workers. The virus can survive outside the body for at least _____ day(s) and can still cause infection in others during that time.

8. _____ is the best option for dealing with hepatitis B.

8. Explain OSHA's Bloodborne Pathogens Standard and the Needlestick Safety and Prevention Act

Multiple Choice

1. The Bloodborne Pathogens Standard is a law that requires that
   (A) Healthcare employers must have a written exposure control plan designed to eliminate or reduce employee exposure to infectious material
   (B) Healthcare employers must only accept patients who are free of bloodborne diseases
   (C) Healthcare employers must charge employees a discounted fee for hepatitis B vaccinations
   (D) Healthcare employers must disclose information about patients' bloodborne diseases to the public

2. Which of the following does OSHA consider a significant exposure?
   (A) PBT is stuck by a needle after a blood draw
   (B) Patient makes a complaint against a PBT
   (C) PBT does not discard their PPE properly
   (D) PBT was recently diagnosed with cancer

3. Which of the following is an example of the type of engineering control required by the Needlestick Safety and Prevention Act?
   (A) An N95 respirator
   (B) An eyewash station
   (C) A hinged or sliding needle sheath
   (D) A sharps container

4. According to OSHA, employers must give all employees, patients, and visitors _____ to use when needed.
   (A) Syringe caps
   (B) Safety Data Sheets (SDS)
   (C) PPE
   (D) Medical charts

5. Why is it important for an employee to report any potential exposures immediately?
   (A) So that the employee can be terminated to avoid infecting others
   (B) To avoid any appearance of negligence on the part of the facility
   (C) To protect the employee's health and the health of others
   (D) So that the employee can warn patients of a possible epidemic

6. In addition to being trained when they are hired, how often do healthcare workers need to take part in in-service training about bloodborne pathogens and updates on any new safety standards?
   (A) Every other year
   (B) Every year
   (C) Every 6 months
   (D) Every 3 months

9. List guidelines for handling equipment and specimens

Matching
Use each letter only once.

1. ____ Clean
2. ____ Dirty
3. ____ Disinfection
4. ____ Sterilization

(A) A cleaning measure that destroys all microorganisms, including those that form spores

(B) A process that destroys most, but not all, pathogens

(C) In health care, objects that have not been contaminated with pathogens

(D) In health care, objects that have been contaminated with pathogens

Multiple Choice

5. Where should specimen tubes and containers be placed for transport?
   (A) In the PBT's pocket
   (B) In a puncture-proof sharps receptacle
   (C) In a plastic zipper bag
   (D) In a biohazard bag

6. After collecting a specimen from a patient, what must the PBT always do before calling the next patient to the drawing station?
   (A) Ask the provider's permission
   (B) Clean and disinfect all surfaces
   (C) Run required tests on the specimen
   (D) Ask the patient to clean everything they touched

7. Where should needles or sharps used in specimen collection be placed?
   (A) In with the specimen
   (B) In a separate biohazard bag
   (C) In the trash
   (D) In a puncture-proof sharps receptacle

10. List employer and employee responsibilities for infection prevention

Short Answer
Read the following and mark ER *for employer or* EE *for employee to show who is responsible for infection prevention.*

1. ____ Immediately report any exposure to infection, blood, or body fluids
2. ____ Provide PPE for use and train how to properly use it
3. ____ Follow all facility policies and procedures
4. ____ Take advantage of the free hepatitis B vaccination
5. ____ Provide continuing in-service education about infection prevention
6. ____ Establish infection prevention procedures and an exposure control plan
7. ____ Follow patient care plans and assignments
8. ____ Participate in continuing in-service education programs covering infection prevention
9. ____ Use PPE as indicated or as appropriate
10. ____ Provide free hepatitis B vaccinations

Please do not copy our workbook. Report violations to legal@hartmanonline.com.

5

Safety Measures for Care Team Members and Patients

1. Discuss the importance of laboratory safety and identify OSHA's categories of common hazards

Fill in the Blank

1. _____ staff members, including _____ _____, are responsible for safety in a facility.

2. Bloodborne pathogens are one significant _____ _____ PBTs may encounter.

3. Physical hazards include poor _____ practices. They also include exposure to _____ or _____ _____.

4. The _____ of chairs for drawing blood, the location of _____ _____ and supplies, and the amount of space at a(n) _____ _____ can all affect safety.

5. Healthcare workers should review and practice safety responses often so that they become _____.

2. Describe regulations related to safety practices in the laboratory and explain the Safety Data Sheet

Matching

1. ____ Work practices
2. ____ Engineering controls
3. ____ PPE
4. ____ Administrative controls

(A) Devices, such as needle sheaths, that prevent workers from coming into contact with hazards

(B) Equipment, such as gloves, used when contact with hazards is likely

(C) Practices, such as using the least caustic cleaning agent, that change how work is done to limit exposure to hazards

(D) Policies and procedures, such as ways to handle blood or body fluids, that employers put in place to limit possible dangers

Multiple Choice

5. What does OSHA's Hazard Communication Standard (*HazCom*) require?
   (A) That signs be placed on patients' doors when they require Transmission-Based Precautions
   (B) That pictograms be used to label potential hazards
   (C) That hazardous chemicals be labeled with detailed descriptions of possible dangers they can cause
   (D) That hazardous chemicals be labeled with the phone number of a poison control center

6. Which of the following is included on a Safety Data Sheet (SDS)?
   (A) Chemical ingredients and dangers
   (B) Correct response to patient abuse
   (C) Fire evacuation procedures
   (D) Safe handling information for blood specimens

7. Employers must
   (A) Keep SDS information confidential from employees
   (B) Terminate employees who do not know how to use an SDS
   (C) Have an SDS for every chemical used
   (D) Edit an SDS if they do not agree with what is listed

3. List safety guidelines for common hazards in laboratory settings

Short Answer

1. According to the CDC, what should be developed in a workplace to avoid danger?

   _____

   _____

2. What should a PBT do if he notices a possible hazard in the workplace?

   _____

   _____

3. List 2 types of chemicals PBTs regularly use on the job.

   _____

   _____

4. Why should dried blood or other body fluids not be scraped off of a surface or floor?

   _____

   _____

   _____

5. What are 2 ways for phlebotomy technicians to protect themselves against radiation exposure?

   _____

   _____

   _____

   _____

6. What should a PBT do about damaged or malfunctioning equipment?

   _____

   _____

   _____

   _____

7. PASS is an acronym that stands for

   _____

   _____

   _____

   _____

8. RACE is an acronym that stands for

   _____

   _____

   _____

   _____

9. Explain the fire safety technique *stop, drop, and roll*.

   _____

   _____

   _____

   _____

Multiple Choice

10. A general guideline to follow during a disaster is to
    (A) Turn off your phone to save battery
    (B) Know where the fire alarms and extinguishers are located
    (C) Carry as many patient files as you can as you leave the facility
    (D) Shout loudly about what is happening so all patients can hear

11. In case of earthquakes it is best to
    (A) Go outside and find the closest tall building
    (B) Shout if trapped under debris
    (C) Get under a sturdy piece of furniture
    (D) Stand on a piece of tall furniture to get as far away from the ground as possible

Name: _____

12. In case of an active shooter it is best to
    (A) Run outside to find a safe place to hide
    (B) Keep your phone ringer on in case police or family members need to contact you
    (C) Secure the door by moving a heavy piece of furniture in front of it
    (D) Find and confront the shooter

4. Discuss measures necessary to protect patients and keep them safe

True or False

1. ____ Taking time to establish an atmosphere of trust with a child can improve safety.

2. ____ If a patient needs a walker, it should be placed directly in front of the phlebotomy chair during the draw.

3. ____ The sharps container can be within reach of a small child as long as the phlebotomist tells the child not to touch it.

4. ____ Elderly patients' limbs and skin may need to be treated more gently than other patients'.

5. ____ A cooperative child may be left unattended at a drawing station for very short periods of time.

6. ____ When drawing blood from a small child at an adult-sized drawing station, it may be safest for the child to be in a parent's lap.

Name: _____

Safety Measures for Care Team Members and Patients

6

Overview of the Human Body

1. Describe body systems and define key anatomical terms

Matching
Use each letter only once.

1. ____ Homeostasis
2. ____ Metabolism
3. ____ Signs
4. ____ Symptoms
5. ____ Organs
6. ____ Tissues
7. ____ Cells
8. ____ Anterior/ventral
9. ____ Distal
10. ____ Medial
11. ____ Inferior
12. ____ Posterior/dorsal
13. ____ Lateral
14. ____ Superior
15. ____ Proximal

(A) Structural unit in the human body that performs a specific function

(B) Physical and chemical processes by which substances are broken down or transformed into energy or products for use by the body

(C) Toward the midline of the body

(D) Subjective information about a person's health

(E) The condition in which all of the body's systems are balanced and are working together to maintain internal stability

(F) To the side, away from the midline of the body

(G) Objective information about a person's health

(H) A group of cells that perform a similar task

(I) Away from the head

(J) Farther away from the torso

(K) Basic structural unit of the body

(L) Closer to the torso

(M) The front of the body or body part

(N) The back of the body or body part

(O) Toward the head

2. Describe the integumentary system

Fill in the Blank

1. The largest organ and system in the body is the _____.

2. Skin prevents _____ to internal organs.

3. Skin also prevents the loss of too much _____, which is essential to life.

4. The skin is also a(n) _____ that feels heat, cold, pain, touch, and pressure.

5. Blood vessels _____, or widen, when the outside temperature is too high.

6. Blood vessels _____, or narrow, when the outside temperature is too cold.

7. Capillaries, the smallest _____ _____ in the body, are located in the _____, which is the inner layer of skin.

8. No blood vessels and only a few nerve endings are located in the _____, which is the outer layer of skin.

9. Allergic reactions can cause integumentary system symptoms. Blood tests for IgE, a type of _____, may be part of allergy diagnosis.

10. A complete blood count (CBC) may also be ordered, as allergies can increase the number of a particular type of _____ _____ in a person's blood.

3. Describe the musculoskeletal system

True or False

1. _____ The body is shaped by muscles, bones, ligaments, tendons, and cartilage.
2. _____ The human body has 215 bones.
3. _____ Bones protect the body's organs.
4. _____ Two bones meet at a joint.
5. _____ Muscles allow movement of body parts.
6. _____ All muscles can be consciously controlled (moved when a person wants to move them).
7. _____ Muscles produce heat for the body.
8. _____ A hinge joint allows movement in all directions.
9. _____ The tissues of the bones are hard and rigid and do not need to receive oxygen or nutrients.
10. _____ Skeletal muscles are attached to bones.
11. _____ Blood tests for certain antibodies may help diagnose arthritis.

4. Describe the nervous system

Multiple Choice

1. The nervous system
   (A) Gives the body shape and structure
   (B) Controls and coordinates body functions
   (C) Is the largest organ in the body
   (D) Pumps blood through the blood vessels to the cells

2. The 2 main parts of the nervous system are
   (A) The cardiovascular system and integumentary system
   (B) Neurons and receptors
   (C) The body and the brain
   (D) The central nervous system and peripheral nervous system

3. The basic unit of the nervous system is the nerve cell, which is also called a(n)
   (A) Synapse
   (B) Receptor
   (C) Neuron
   (D) Ossicle

4. The peripheral nervous system deals with the outer part of the body via the
   (A) Brain
   (B) Cerebrum
   (C) Nerves
   (D) Right hemisphere

5. What cushions the brain and spinal cord against injury?
   (A) The nerves
   (B) The spinal column
   (C) The brainstem
   (D) Cerebrospinal fluid

6. The _____ is the part of the brain that controls thinking, speech, and voluntary muscles.
   (A) Brainstem
   (B) Cerebellum
   (C) Cerebral cortex
   (D) Right hemisphere

7. The left hemisphere of the brain controls
   (A) The left side of the body
   (B) The right side of the body
   (C) Both sides of the body
   (D) Memory

8. The brainstem controls
   (A) Smooth movements
   (B) Breathing and swallowing
   (C) Jerky movements
   (D) Emotions and speech

9. The nerve pathways in the spinal cord conduct messages between
   (A) The heart and the blood
   (B) The cerebrum and cerebellum
   (C) The brain and the body
   (D) The muscles and the bones

10. The central nervous system is made up of
    (A) The brain and spinal cord
    (B) Muscles and bones
    (C) Neurons and receptors
    (D) The heart and lungs

Short Answer

11. List the 5 sense organs of the body.

   _____

   _____

   _____

   _____

12. Which part of the eye contains cells that respond to light and send a message to the brain so that a person can see?

   _____

13. List the 3 parts of the ear.

   _____

   _____

   _____

14. Why may a provider order blood tests when diagnosing a possible stroke or a nervous system disorder such as Parkinson's disease?

   _____

   _____

   _____

   _____

5. Describe the respiratory system

True or False

1. ____ Respiration occurs in the lungs.
2. ____ Expiration is breathing in.
3. ____ The respiratory system brings oxygen into the body and eliminates carbon dioxide from the body.
4. ____ The larynx is also called the windpipe.
5. ____ Oxygen and carbon dioxide are exchanged between the alveoli and the capillaries.
6. ____ The pleura is a 2-layered membrane that covers the lungs.
7. ____ The pharynx divides into the right bronchus and left bronchus.
8. ____ The pulmonary vein carries oxygen-saturated blood to the left side of the heart.

Multiple Choice

9. What is located between the layers of the pleura?
   (A) The alveoli
   (B) Lubricating fluid
   (C) The pulmonary veins
   (D) Special tissue that protects the respiratory system from pathogens

10. In adult patients, blood gas testing is usually performed
    (A) On blood from capillaries
    (B) On blood from venules
    (C) On blood from veins
    (D) On blood from arteries

6. Describe the urinary system

Short Answer

1. List 2 functions of the urinary system.

   _____

   _____

   _____

   _____

34

2. What are the parts of the urinary system?
   _____
   _____
   _____
   _____

3. Where are waste products and excess water filtered from the blood?
   _____

4. What path does urine follow from the kidneys to leave the body?
   _____
   _____
   _____

5. What is the name of the series of blood tests that may be ordered to evaluate kidney health?
   _____

6. What task related to the diagnosis of urinary tract infection may be assigned to a phlebotomy technician?
   _____
   _____

7. Describe the gastrointestinal system

Crossword

Across

3. Process of expelling wastes (made up of the waste products of food and fluids) that are not absorbed into the cells

4. Involuntary contractions that move food into the stomach from the esophagus

6. Transfer of nutrients from the intestines to the cells

7. Semisolid material made up of water, solid waste material, bacteria, and mucus that passes through the rectum and out of the body

Down

1. Process of preparing food physically and chemically so that it can be absorbed into the cells

2. Semiliquid substance created by the breaking down of food in the stomach

5. Muscular pouch located in the upper left part of the abdominal cavity

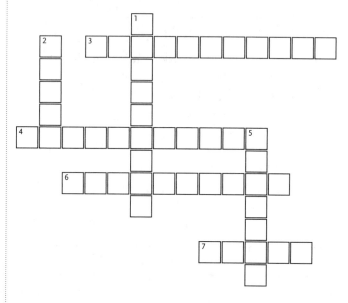

Short Answer

8. What parts and organs of the body are considered accessories to digestion?
   _____
   _____
   _____
   _____
   _____

9. What CLIA waived test related to the digestive system may be performed by a phlebotomy technician or other certified healthcare worker?
   _____
   _____

10. What part of the body does a *hepatic function panel* relate to?
    _____

Name: _____

8. Describe the endocrine system

Fill in the Blank

1. The endocrine system is made up of _____ in different areas of the body.

2. _____ are chemical substances created by the body that control numerous body functions.

3. Three hormones secreted by the pituitary gland are _____ _____, _____ _____, and _____.

4. The thyroid gland, which is located in the _____, produces thyroid hormone, which regulates _____.

5. The parathyroid glands secrete a hormone that regulates the body's use of _____.

6. Insulin, a hormone that works to move _____ (natural sugar) from the blood and into the cells for energy for the body, is secreted by the _____.

7. The hormone adrenaline regulates muscle power, heart rate, blood pressure, and energy levels during _____ situations or _____.

8. Patients with diagnosed diabetes may _____ their own blood to determine how much _____ is present.

9. Glucose challenge tests and glucose tolerance tests are commonly performed during _____ to check for _____ _____.

9. Describe the reproductive system

Multiple Choice

1. The reproductive system allows humans to
   (A) Move and speak
   (B) Create human life
   (C) Think logically
   (D) Fight disease

2. The male and female sex glands are the
   (A) Adrenals
   (B) Ureters
   (C) Gonads
   (D) Urethras

3. The hormone needed for male reproductive organs to function properly is
   (A) Sperm
   (B) Adrenaline
   (C) Estrogen
   (D) Testosterone

4. The gonads in females are called
   (A) Ovaries
   (B) Eggs
   (C) Testicles
   (D) Sex cells

5. The female reproductive cycle is maintained by the hormones
   (A) Estrogen and progesterone
   (B) Adrenaline and progesterone
   (C) Testosterone and ADH
   (D) Insulin and testosterone

6. Pregnancy tests detect the presence of the hormone
   (A) Oxytocin
   (B) Prolactin
   (C) hCG
   (D) Insulin

10. Describe the immune and lymphatic systems

Fill in the Blank

1. The immune system protects the body from disease-causing _____, viruses, and microorganisms.

2. _____ immunity protects the body from disease in general.

3. _____ immunity protects against a disease that is invading the body at a given time.

4. The lymphatic system removes excess _____ and waste products from the tissues.

5. _____ is a clear yellowish fluid that carries disease-fighting cells. The cells are called _____.

Short Answer

6. List 3 ways the body protects itself against disease in general.

   _____
   _____
   _____
   _____
   _____

7. What are 2 ways a person can gain acquired immunity?

   _____
   _____
   _____
   _____

8. Why is muscle activity important to the function of the lymphatic system?

   _____
   _____
   _____
   _____

7

The Circulatory System in Depth

1. Describe the circulatory system and the structure and function of the heart

Multiple Choice

1. What functions as the pump of the circulatory system?
   (A) Heart
   (B) Lungs
   (C) Lymph
   (D) Blood

2. What structure divides the sides of the heart?
   (A) The epicardium
   (B) The aortic valve
   (C) The septum
   (D) The ventricles

3. What do the heart's valves do?
   (A) Trigger the pumping action of the heart
   (B) Keep blood flowing in the correct direction
   (C) Move electrical signals through the heart
   (D) Receive nerve impulses

Fill in the Blank

4. The top of the heart is known as the _____ and the bottom of the heart is known as the _____.

5. The atria are the 2 _____ chambers of the heart. The 2 _____ chambers are called ventricles.

6. The _____ ventricle pumps oxygenated blood out of the heart via the _____.

7. The back-and-forth action between the upper and lower chambers allows the chambers to _____ with blood before they contract to _____ the blood.

8. The 4 major valves of the heart are the _____ valve, the _____ valve, the _____ valve, and the _____ valve.

2. Explain the cardiac conduction system

Matching
Use each letter only once.

1. ____ Atrioventricular junction
2. ____ Bundle of His
3. ____ Purkinje fibers
4. ____ Cardiac conduction system
5. ____ Bundle branches
6. ____ Sinoatrial node
7. ____ Atrioventricular node

(A) The heart's electrical signal (impulse) travels here from the atrioventricular node.

(B) The impulse is first carried to the walls of the ventricles through this part of the conduction system.

(C) This is the main pacemaker of the heart, where the heart's electrical signal (impulse) begins.

(D) The heart's electrical signal (impulse) travels here from the SA node.

(E) The impulse travels here from the AV junction; it is also called the *AV bundle*.

(F) The impulse follows these small branches as they divide from the bundle branches.

(G) The network of tissue in the heart that carries electrical signals that prompt heartbeats

3. Describe blood vessels

True or False

1. ____ The aorta is the largest vein in the body.
2. ____ Arteries have thicker walls than veins.
3. ____ At any given time about 70% of the body's blood is found in the veins.
4. ____ There are valves inside veins that help keep blood moving in the right direction.
5. ____ A pulse can be felt in both veins and arteries.
6. ____ Capillary beds carry deoxygenated blood from the heart to the lungs.
7. ____ To *palpate* means to listen with a stethoscope.

Matching
Use each letter only once.

8. ____ Tunica media
9. ____ Artery
10. ____ Capillary bed
11. ____ Tunica intima
12. ____ Pulmonary circuit
13. ____ Vein
14. ____ Inferior vena cava
15. ____ Tunica adventitia
16. ____ Systemic circuit
17. ____ Superior vena cava

(A) A blood vessel that carries blood away from the heart

(B) Areas where exchanges of oxygen and carbon dioxide, and nutrients and waste products, take place

(C) Large vein that carries blood to the heart from the legs and trunk

(D) Large vein that carries blood from the arms, head, and neck to the heart

(E) The outer layer of veins or arteries

(F) The inner layer of veins or arteries

(G) The middle layer of veins or arteries

(H) A blood vessel that carries blood toward the heart

(I) The circulation of blood between the heart and the rest of the body (except the lungs)

(J) The circulation of blood between the heart and the lungs

4. Describe the components of blood

Multiple Choice

1. Which of the following is a type of white blood cell?
   (A) Erythrocyte
   (B) Thrombocyte
   (C) Fibrinogen
   (D) Lymphocyte

2. What is plasma mostly made up of?
   (A) Water
   (B) Oxygen
   (C) Lymph
   (D) Minerals

3. The disc-like shape of erythrocytes allows them to
   (A) Plug up an injury and stop bleeding
   (B) Fight pathogens
   (C) Bend to fit into blood vessels of all sizes
   (D) Carry oxygen

4. What is the name of the large cells that fragment into platelets?
   (A) Monocytes
   (B) Megakaryocytes
   (C) Eosinophils
   (D) Granulocytes

5. A complete blood count that includes a count of each type of white blood cell is called
   (A) A complete blood count +
   (B) A complete blood count with calculation
   (C) A fully complete blood count
   (D) A complete blood count with differential

Name: _____

6. Many types of blood cells originate in the
   (A) Bone marrow
   (B) Spinal column
   (C) Pancreas
   (D) Liver

7. The most numerous type of white blood cell is the
   (A) Neutrophil
   (B) B cell
   (C) T cell
   (D) Basophil

8. How do macrophages protect the body against foreign microorganisms?
   (A) By binding to antigens
   (B) By "eating" them, or surrounding them and breaking them up
   (C) By forming a barrier that does not allow them to enter the body
   (D) By poisoning them

9. Which cells work together to produce antibodies that help the immune system respond to infection?
   (A) Erythrocytes and leukocytes
   (B) Megakaryocytes and erythrocytes
   (C) Basophils and antigens
   (D) B cells and T cells

10. What is the name of a condition in which a person has either too few red blood cells or too little hemoglobin in the blood?
    (A) Sickle cell disease
    (B) Leukemia
    (C) Anemia
    (D) Hemophilia

5. Explain the ABO blood group system and the Rh factor

Short Answer

1. What are the antigens most commonly present on red blood cells? Do all people have the same antigens?

   _____

   _____

   _____

2. What types of antibodies does a person with type O blood have?

   _____

   _____

3. What antigens, antibodies, and proteins are present on a red blood cell of a person with AB+ blood?

   _____

   _____

   _____

4. What happens the first time the blood of a person who is Rh-negative is exposed to Rh-positive blood? What may happen if the person's blood is exposed to Rh-positive blood a second time?

   _____

   _____

   _____

   _____

   _____

5. Why are pregnant women tested for blood type and Rh factor?

   _____

   _____

   _____

   _____

True or False

6. _____ People with O– blood can receive a transfusion from anyone with any blood type.

7. _____ One reason to carefully identify patients and label blood specimens is that even a small amount of the wrong blood type can cause health problems or death.

8. _____ A person with type A blood has anti-A antibodies.

9. ____ People with AB+ blood are known as *universal recipients*.

10. ____ A+ and O+ are the two most common blood types.

6. Describe the qualities of arterial, venous, and capillary blood

Short Answer
For exercises 1–10, write A *for arterial blood,* V *for venous blood, or* B *for both.*

1. ____ Often shown as blue in illustrations and may appear blue under the skin, but is not actually blue

2. ____ May spurt or spray from a wound due to the pressure created by the beating heart

3. ____ Contains hemoglobin

4. ____ In most cases, is carrying oxygen

5. ____ Is very dark red

6. ____ Is moving toward the heart

7. ____ Must be drawn from the body using some amount of force (e.g., from a syringe or evacuated tube)

8. ____ Is bright red

9. ____ May be deoxygenated

10. ____ Can be found in capillaries

11. Capillary blood is a color that is between the colors of venous blood and arterial blood. Why is this?

_____

_____

7. Discuss hemostasis and coagulation and related conditions

Matching
Use each letter only once.

1. ____ Plasmin
2. ____ Vasoconstriction
3. ____ Thrombosis
4. ____ Hemostatic plug
5. ____ Hemostasis
6. ____ Fibrin
7. ____ Thrombin
8. ____ Primary hemostasis
9. ____ Fibrinolysis
10. ____ Enzyme
11. ____ Secondary hemostasis
12. ____ Fibrinogen
13. ____ Coagulation cascade

(A) A protein that forms a mesh with platelets to stop bleeding when injury occurs

(B) A substance in the body that speeds up a specific reaction

(C) The stopping of a flow of blood

(D) The protein that is turned into fibrin when injury occurs

(E) The breaking down of fibrin as an injury heals

(F) The mesh of fibrin and activated platelets formed at an injury site

(G) An enzyme that plays a vital role in breaking apart fibrin as an injury heals

(H) The stage of hemostasis that concludes with the formation of the hemostatic plug

(I) Reaction to injury in a blood vessel causing narrowing of tissue at the injury site

(J) The first stage of hemostasis, concluding with the formation of a platelet plug

(K) An enzyme in plasma that controls platelet response

(L) The formation of a clot within a blood vessel

(M) A series of changes in the body to prevent blood loss while also avoiding unnecessary and dangerous excessive clotting

Name: _____

Labeling/Short Answer

For exercises 14–16, label what is shown in the picture, then write a brief description of each pictured stage of hemostasis.

14.

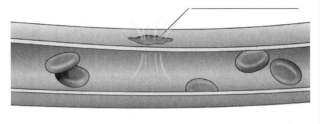

_____
_____
_____
_____

15.

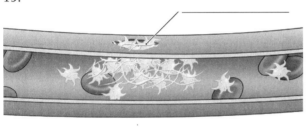

_____
_____
_____
_____

16.

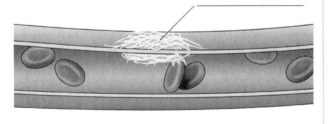

_____
_____
_____
_____

Multiple Choice

17. A person who has hemophilia
    (A) Is prone to excessive blood clotting and is treated with anticoagulants
    (B) Is prone to excessive bleeding and is treated with infusions of clotting factors
    (C) Is at high risk for pulmonary embolism
    (D) Is likely to have abnormal heart rhythms

18. Anticoagulants are drugs that
    (A) Speed up blood clotting
    (B) Provide the body with clotting factors that are missing
    (C) Slow down blood clotting
    (D) Regulate the heart's rhythm

19. A phlebotomy technician should ensure that bleeding has stopped before a patient leaves the drawing station
    (A) Only when the PBT performed capillary puncture
    (B) Only when the PBT performed venipuncture
    (C) Only if the patient has hemophilia or is taking an anticoagulant
    (D) After every blood draw

Short Answer

20. Describe what happens to blood that is collected in a tube without an anticoagulant additive. How long does this take?

_____
_____
_____
_____

21. What happens when a specimen tube is spun in a centrifuge?

_____
_____
_____
_____

22. What is the liquid portion called in a centrifuged blood specimen that does not contain an anticoagulant?

   _____

23. What is the liquid portion called in a centrifuged blood specimen that contains an anticoagulant? What does it include that is not found in the liquid portion of a clotted specimen?

   _____
   _____
   _____
   _____

24. What is the name of the layer between the liquid and solid portions of a plasma specimen? What does it contain?

   _____
   _____
   _____
   _____

25. Why is it important for PBTs to know the difference between different types of blood specimens (e.g., plasma, serum, whole blood)?

   _____
   _____
   _____
   _____

8

Preparing for Specimen Collection

1. Discuss venipuncture and capillary puncture and identify different types of specimens collected by phlebotomy technicians

Fill in the Blank

1. Most blood specimens are collected by _____, or the puncture of a(n) _____.

2. Point-of-care tests generally require that blood from a(n) _____ _____ be placed directly onto a test strip that is inserted into a machine for _____.

3. In adults and in children over _____ year(s) old, capillary puncture is performed on the _____.

4. Many blood collection tubes contain _____ _____ that act to prepare the blood for testing.

5. A test commonly performed on newborns requires that capillary blood be dripped onto _____ _____.

6. The primary job of a(n) _____ is to collect blood specimens for analysis.

7. Tubes used to collect venipuncture specimens are _____ than those used to collect capillary specimens.

8. For infants, capillary puncture is performed at the _____.

9. Blood culture testing involves collecting samples in bottles that allow any _____ in the blood to multiply.

2. Describe the importance of avoiding errors before and during specimen collection

Short Answer

1. How might careful work by a phlebotomy technician promote good health for a patient? How might mistakes made by a phlebotomy technician harm a patient's health?

_____
_____
_____
_____
_____
_____
_____
_____
_____
_____
_____
_____
_____
_____
_____

2. What is the term for errors that happen before a specimen is tested?

_____
_____

3. How should a PBT check a patient's name to be sure it matches the requisition?

_____
_____
_____

4. What else is part of properly identifying a patient?

_____
_____

5. List 3 common requirements that patients may be asked to meet before a blood test.

_____
_____
_____
_____

Place a check mark (✓) next to the items that are examples of preanalytical errors.

6. _____ Using smaller collection tubes for pediatric patients than for adult patients

7. _____ Not mixing a specimen properly

8. _____ Not using correct technique during a blood draw

9. _____ Identifying a patient by 2 unique identifiers

10. _____ Making sure a patient has been fasting if fasting is required

11. _____ Not filling collection tubes in the correct order

12. _____ Not filling tubes to the fill line

13. _____ Checking the requisition and using the tubes ordered for each test

14. _____ Not handling or transporting specimens properly.

3. Discuss common blood specimen collection systems and identify equipment used for venipuncture and capillary puncture

Matching
Use each letter only once.

1. _____ Bevel
2. _____ Winged collection set
3. _____ Syringe transfer device
4. _____ Evacuated tube system
5. _____ Flange
6. _____ Hub
7. _____ Gauge
8. _____ Multisample needle
9. _____ Syringe
10. _____ Shaft
11. _____ Lumen
12. _____ Evacuated tube

(A) The angled opening of a phlebotomy needle

(B) A needle, holder, and vacuum tube used together to collect blood specimens by venipuncture

(C) Indication of the size of a phlebotomy needle; a measurement of the width of the needle's opening

(D) The threaded area at the base of a phlebotomy needle that can be screwed into a holder or syringe

(E) A double-sided needle used in phlebotomy; one side pierces the patient's skin and the other punctures the stoppers of collection tubes

(F) A device similar to a tube holder, used to safely transfer blood from a syringe into evacuated tubes

Name: _____

(G) The hollow space inside a phlebotomy needle

(H) A phlebotomy needle with flaps at the base, attached to a length of tubing, which may be used either with a tube holder or a syringe; commonly called a *butterfly needle*

(I) A tubular device with a plunger that, when pulled, acts to draw in fluid (e.g., blood)

(J) The plastic ridge or edge of a tube holder; can be used for leverage when inserting or changing collection tubes

(K) Tubes emptied of air during the manufacturing process and designed to draw in the exact amount of blood needed for a specimen

(L) The long, hollow tube part of a needle

True or False

13. _____ Higher gauge numbers mean wider (larger) needles.

14. _____ Needles for blood collection have built-in mechanisms to protect against accidental needlesticks.

15. _____ The most common needle gauge for adult venipuncture is 21.

16. _____ The gauge of a needle is printed in large numbers on the hub of the needle.

17. _____ Larger collection tubes create a stronger pull on the patient's vein.

18. _____ Blood culture collections are done with butterfly assemblies.

19. _____ Winged collection sets are often used on patients who have large, easy-to-access veins.

20. _____ A syringe always puts greater pressure on a patient's veins than an evacuated tube.

21. _____ The same size of collection tube is used for all venipuncture draws on adults.

Fill in the Blank

22. New gloves must be used for _____.

23. An allergy to _____ should be noted on a requisition form, but it is a good idea to ask a patient and use _____ gloves if needed.

24. The antiseptic most commonly used to prepare for venipuncture is a 70% _____ _____ _____.

25. An antiseptic often used during blood culture preparation is _____.

26. Antiseptics containing _____ should not be used on patients who have an allergy to it or to _____.

27. A(n) _____ restricts the return of _____ blood below the area where it is applied.

28. _____ is applied to the puncture site immediately following venipuncture. Applying _____ to it will help stop the flow of blood.

29. Standard adhesive or self-adhesive wrap style _____ are placed over the gauze after venipuncture. _____ is a common brand name for the wrap style.

30. Electronic vein-finding devices or _____ _____ may be used to assist in locating a patient's veins.

Multiple Choice

31. Which of these lists includes equipment used both during venipuncture and during capillary puncture?
    (A) Antiseptic, gauze, evacuated tube, lancet
    (B) Butterfly assembly, tourniquet, microcollection tube, bandage
    (C) Antiseptic, gauze, gloves, bandage
    (D) Gloves, antiseptic, microcollection tube, evacuated tube

32. The volume of liquid a capillary collection tube can hold is generally
    (A) 125–600 microliters
    (B) 125–600 milliliters
    (C) 125–600 cubic centimeters
    (D) 125–600 ounces

33. Which of the following is true of microcollection tubes?
    (A) They are emptied of air during manufacture.
    (B) They have rubber stoppers so they can be changed out easily.
    (C) They may have a spout or straw-like attachment to make collection easier.
    (D) They are always sealed with a clay-like substance.

34. What anticoagulant is sometimes used to treat capillary tubes?
    (A) Eliquis
    (B) Heparin
    (C) Warfarin
    (D) Acetylsalicylic acid

35. Adhesive bandages are never put on patients who are
    (A) Elderly
    (B) Allergic to latex
    (C) Taking anticoagulant medications
    (D) Infants or toddlers

36. What equipment may be used to improve blood flow before capillary puncture?
    (A) A warming pack
    (B) A Venoscope
    (C) A tourniquet
    (D) An ice pack

37. Which of the following describes a common type of lancet?
    (A) Has a hub that a retractable needle is screwed into
    (B) Is pressed against the patient's skin to activate
    (C) Is sterilized and reused
    (D) Has an exposed blade that slices the patient's skin

4. Identify additives to blood specimens and describe the color coding of collection tubes

Crossword

Across

4. Tubes without anticoagulants are sometimes called this.
6. General term for chemicals in collection tubes that prepare the blood for analysis
8. Substances studied in diagnostic tests

Down

1. Part of the collection tube that is color-coded based on the chemical in the tube
2. A complete blood count test is performed on this type of blood.
3. Tubes that contain anticoagulants are sometimes called this.
5. A fill line or arrow on a tube label indicates the _____ of the tube.
7. Specimens for serum testing must be allowed to do this before testing.

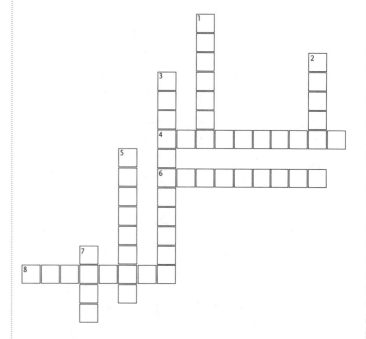

Name: _____

True or False

9. ____ Different anticoagulant additives act in different ways.

10. ____ Some collection tubes contain a gel that, when a specimen is centrifuged, creates a barrier between the liquid and solid components.

11. ____ Blood in a collection tube is mixed with the additive by shaking it vigorously for 5–10 seconds.

12. ____ Tan-topped tubes are usually used for coagulation studies.

13. ____ Specimens can be mixed with tube additives any time within 15 minutes of collection.

14. ____ Tube labels list additives contained in the tube.

15. ____ Tube stoppers are identical no matter the manufacturer of the tube.

Matching

Letters may be used more than once.

16. ____ May contain acid citrate dextrose (ACD) or sodium polyanethol sulfonate (SPS)

17. ____ Most often used for routine chemistry tests

18. ____ Contains an additive to prevent glycolysis

19. ____ Often referred to as *citrate tubes*

20. ____ Used for hematology studies, including complete blood count

21. ____ Contains EDTA

22. ____ Contains an anticoagulant that is reversible; may be used to study clotting time

23. ____ Certified to be free of trace elements

24. ____ Contains the anticoagulant heparin

25. ____ Contains the same anticoagulant as tubes with white or pink stoppers

26. ____ May contain sodium oxalate, potassium oxalate, or EDTA as an anticoagulant, along with sodium fluoride

27. ____ May be used for paternity testing

(A) Light blue stopper

(B) Green stopper

(C) Lavender stopper

(D) Gray stopper

(E) Yellow stopper

(F) Royal blue stopper

5. List the order in which collection tubes must be filled (order of draw)

1. Why do venipuncture tubes need to be filled in a specific order?

   _____
   _____
   _____
   _____
   _____

2. List the CLSI order of draw for venipuncture.

   _____
   _____
   _____
   _____
   _____
   _____
   _____
   _____
   _____
   _____
   _____
   _____

Name: _____

3. A PBT needs to draw a lavender tube, a light blue tube, and a green tube. In what order should they be drawn?

   _____
   _____

4. A patient needs a blood culture and also needs a light blue tube drawn. What will the PBT draw first?

   _____
   _____

5. Why is order of draw different for capillary collections?

   _____
   _____
   _____
   _____
   _____
   _____

6. What is the order of draw for capillary collections?

   _____
   _____
   _____
   _____

7. What is a discard tube? What type of tube is best to use as a discard?

   _____
   _____
   _____
   _____
   _____

8. What should a PBT do if a requisition requires an unfamiliar tube?

   _____
   _____
   _____
   _____

6. Describe considerations for timing of blood draws

Scenarios
Read each scenario below and then answer the questions about timing considerations.

1. PBT Alina has requisitions for 3 patients. One is marked *stat*. The other 2 are routine. One of the patients in for routine testing has been fasting. The other has not been. In what order should Alina call the patients?

   _____
   _____
   _____
   _____
   _____
   _____
   _____
   _____

2. Angelica is a PBT at a women's clinic. A patient is in for a glucose tolerance test. Angelica drew her blood before she drank the glucose beverage. Angelica sees that it is now time to do the second blood draw, but she just received a requisition marked *ASAP*. Can Angelica do the blood draw for the glucose tolerance test before she does the test marked *ASAP*? Why or why not?

   _____
   _____
   _____
   _____

Name: _____

3. Mr. Kenenisa took his medication about an hour ago. He has an order to measure trough medication level. When should PBT Carlos draw blood to perform this test? Can he do that now?

_____
_____
_____
_____
_____
_____
_____

4. Ana is a PBT at a hospital. She needs to test Mrs. Roland for peak medication levels. Does it matter for the timing of the test whether Mrs. Roland receives the medication by IV or by mouth? Why or why not?

_____
_____
_____
_____
_____
_____

7. Discuss the steps required to properly identify patients and specimens

Short Answer
Place a check mark (✓) next to the items that describe problems that can result from incorrect identification of a patient.

1. ____ Illness or death due to transfusion or medication administration
2. ____ Transmission of a bloodborne disease from an infected needle
3. ____ Inaccurate test results because tubes were drawn in the wrong order
4. ____ Inconvenience and pain caused by additional blood draws
5. ____ Painful hematomas or nerve damage
6. ____ Inaccurate diagnosis or treatment
7. ____ Increased costs due to repeated testing or incorrect care
8. ____ Possible legal action against the phlebotomist and/or the facility

Fill in the Blank

9. The standard information used to identify a patient is _____ _____ and _____ _____ _____.

10. A patient's _____ _____ at a hospital is not uniquely identifying and should not be used to confirm identity.

11. CLSI recommends that patients should both _____ and _____ their first and last names and speak their _____ _____ _____.

12. Information about identity provided by the patient must be checked against the _____/specimen labels and the patient's _____, if used.

13. A patient's _____ must be on their _____ to be considered a valid form of identification. It cannot be on a hospital bed rail or on a bedside table, for example.

14. If a family member or nurse helps to confirm the identity of a nonverbal or unresponsive patient, the PBT must document the _____ of the individual who helps.

15. Before a patient leaves a drawing station or a PBT leaves a patient's bedside, the PBT should ask the patient to _____ that name/date of birth on the collection tubes is _____.

Short Answer

16. List 3 situations in which an identification error is more likely to occur. What is the best way to prevent these errors?

_____
_____
_____
_____

8. Describe preparations for the safe collection of blood specimens

Short Answer

1. When must a PBT wear gloves during a blood draw?

_____
_____
_____

2. Where should the sharps container be while a PBT is drawing blood?

_____
_____
_____

3. When is a sharps container considered to be full?

_____
_____
_____

4. What can a PBT do to be ready for unexpected challenges before they arise?

_____
_____
_____

9. List preparations for protecting the integrity of specimens during collection and transportation

True or False

1. _____ With some routine blood specimens it is not important to protect the tubes against jostling or rough handling.

2. _____ When testing for bilirubin, the specimen must be placed in an ice slurry.

3. _____ A PBT should know any special handling requirements before completing a draw so that any necessary equipment is available right away.

4. _____ Specimens that must be protected from light may be drawn in a clear tube and then placed in a light-protected specimen bag.

5. _____ If specimens are not kept at the correct temperature, test results may not be accurate.

6. _____ If a PBT is not sure how a specimen should be handled, she should keep it cold and protect it from light.

10. Discuss furniture and accessories necessary to a phlebotomy station

Multiple Choice

1. How are blood draws usually done on young pediatric patients in a general (i.e., nonpediatric) setting?
   (A) In a standard phlebotomy chair with no adjustments
   (B) In a bariatric phlebotomy chair
   (C) With the patient supine on an examination table
   (D) With a parent or guardian holding the child

Name: _____

2. What furniture or accessory should be available for use when performing a blood draw on a patient who has a history of fainting?
   (A) A bariatric phlebotomy chair
   (B) A foam wedge to keep the patient upright
   (C) A reclining chair or a flat surface to lie on
   (D) A neck brace to prevent the patient from hitting his head if he faints

3. What must be done with devices such as arm wedges that are used with more than one patient?
   (A) They must have disposable paper covers.
   (B) They must be sterilized between patients.
   (C) They must be rinsed with soap and water between patients.
   (D) They must be sanitized between patients.

4. If a blood pressure cuff is used as a tourniquet, it should be inflated
   (A) Until the patient says it feels tight
   (B) Until the PBT can barely slip 2 fingers under the cuff
   (C) Until the blood pressure reading is just above the patient's systolic reading
   (D) Until the blood pressure reading is just below the patient's diastolic reading

5. In a typical outpatient laboratory, a phlebotomy station usually has a standard phlebotomy chair, a bariatric phlebotomy chair, and
   (A) An examination table
   (B) A cart or cabinet for supplies
   (C) A pediatric phlebotomy chair
   (D) A reclining chair that looks like a dentist's chair

6. A bariatric chair is made to accommodate patients who
   (A) Are obese
   (B) Are under 12 years old
   (C) Are prone to seizures
   (D) Are anxious about blood draws

7. Which of the following statements about the work of a phlebotomist makes ergonomics especially important in the phlebotomist's workspace?
   (A) Phlebotomists work with patients of all ages and conditions.
   (B) Phlebotomy is repetitive work and can cause strain to the PBT's body.
   (C) Phlebotomists must identify patients carefully for every blood draw.
   (D) Phlebotomists must handle specimens correctly to ensure accurate test results.

9
Collecting Blood Specimens by Venipuncture

1. Review how blood tests are ordered

Matching
Use each letter only once.

1. ____ Special requirements
2. ____ Requisition
3. ____ Laboratory information system (LIS)
4. ____ Diagnosis codes
5. ____ Accession number
6. ____ Tests

(A) Electronic records that integrate every part of the laboratory testing process

(B) May include fasting, basal state, specific collection times

(C) Listed based on provider orders; listing may include tubes to be used for each

(D) May be listed on the requisition; discussion is beyond scope of practice for PBTs

(E) Paper or electronic record of tests ordered for a specific patient

(F) Identifier related to all specimens on a requisition; allows the specimen to be traced through each stage of the testing process

2. Identify the most common venipuncture blood tests

Short Answer

1. What are 3 reasons blood tests may be ordered?

   _____

   _____

   _____

2. What is a test panel?

   _____

   _____

   _____

   _____

3. What tests are usually included in a lipid panel?

   _____

   _____

   _____

   _____

4. What tube may be used when a stat metabolic or lipid panel is ordered?

   _____

5. What tube is used for a complete blood count? Why is this type of tube needed?

   _____

   _____

   _____

3. Describe appropriate tourniquet use

Fill in the Blank

1. A tourniquet is applied _____ to _____ inches above the puncture site.

2. Since venipuncture is usually performed inside the _____, the tourniquet is first applied to a patient's _____.

3. Constriction from the tourniquet causes the veins below to become fuller than usual, making them easier to _____ and _____.

4. Tourniquets should be applied in such a way that they can be _____ quickly and easily.

5. A tourniquet is used to aid in vein _____ and then _____.

6. A tourniquet must be left on for no longer than _____ _____.

True or False

7. _____ Extended tourniquet use can cause discomfort and can affect test results.

8. _____ When a tourniquet is left in place too long, blood specimens may have fewer blood cells than usual.

9. _____ When venipuncture is performed on the back of the hand, the tourniquet is placed directly on the wrist.

10. _____ For patients with fragile skin, a tourniquet may be placed over clothing or the patient's arm wrapped in gauze before the tourniquet is applied.

11. _____ Hemolysis is the destruction of red blood cells and it can result from excessive tourniquet use.

12. _____ If a tourniquet must be released due to excessive time on the patient's arm, the PBT must wait 10 minutes before reapplying the tourniquet to the same arm.

Short Answer

13. For every *false* answer in exercises 7–12, create a true statement.

_____

_____

_____

_____

_____

_____

_____

_____

_____

4. Identify appropriate sites for venipuncture

Multiple Choice

1. Where on the body is venipuncture most often done?
   (A) On the dorsal aspect of the hand
   (B) On the wrist
   (C) In the antecubital fossa
   (D) On the lateral plantar surface of the foot

2. Which of the following is a reason the median cubital vein is the first choice for venipuncture?
   (A) It always produces good blood flow.
   (B) It is never painful to puncture.
   (C) It is easy to reach.
   (D) It is well anchored and not close to arteries or nerves.

3. Which vein should be the last choice for venipuncture?
   (A) The cephalic vein
   (B) The basilic vein
   (C) The lateral antebrachial vein
   (D) The medial antebrachial vein

4. What is the best way to find a good vein for venipuncture?
   (A) By palpation
   (B) By sight
   (C) By asking the patient which vein is best
   (D) By probing with the needle

5. How should a healthy vein feel?
   (A) Ropy and dense
   (B) Hard and bumpy
   (C) Soft and movable
   (D) Springy and uniform

Name: _____

6. If a patient's veins are located relatively deep under the skin, the PBT should
   (A) Insert the needle at a lower angle
   (B) Insert the needle at a higher angle
   (C) Use a longer needle
   (D) Use a shorter needle

7. Why should a patient not pump their fist while the PBT looks for a vein?
   (A) It will make the puncture uncomfortable.
   (B) Pumping the fist with a tourniquet in place can cause the vein to pop.
   (C) It can cause hemoconcentration and/or hemolysis.
   (D) It can cause the arm to move, which makes it harder to find the vein.

8. When is it appropriate to use a vein in the hand for venipuncture?
   (A) When a vein in the inner elbow cannot be found or cannot be used
   (B) Any time the PBT is using a butterfly needle
   (C) Any time a specimen is being drawn for blood culture
   (D) When the patient is a young child

Place a check mark (✓) next to correct actions when selecting a venipuncture site.

9. ____ Avoiding locations where arteries and nerves may accidentally be hit

10. ____ Checking both arms for a better choice before using the basilic vein

11. ____ Using a vein in the foot when a suitable vein cannot be found in the antecubital fossa

12. ____ Planning to insert the needle at a steeper angle if the vein seems deep in the patient's arm

13. ____ Make patient safety the first priority and also consider the patient's comfort

14. ____ Always using the site a patient says is best

Scenarios

15. PBT Corey has visually inspected and palpated the antecubital fossa on both of Mrs. Martin's arms. She is having a hard time finding a good vein. Are there techniques Corey could use to improve her chance of finding a vein?

   _____
   _____
   _____
   _____
   _____

16. After trying several different techniques to find a vein, Corey asks Mrs. Martin if she can remember where she has had blood drawn successfully before. Mrs. Martin says that her blood is usually drawn from the back of her hand. She says she does not mind having that done. What should Corey do?

   _____
   _____
   _____
   _____
   _____

17. Later in the day, Corey mentions to a coworker that she had an especially hard time finding a good vein on a patient earlier. The coworker suggests that next time Corey should try flicking or slapping the inside of the patient's elbow. Is this a good suggestion? Why or why not?

   _____
   _____
   _____
   _____
   _____

5. Describe the proper cleaning of a venipuncture site

True or False

1. _____ Current CLSI standards say that a venipuncture site must be cleaned in concentric circles.

2. _____ Blowing on a venipuncture site after cleaning is an effective way to dry the antiseptic agent.

3. _____ Sites for blood culture specimen collection must be cleaned more thoroughly than sites for other tests.

4. _____ Povidone-iodine should not be used on patients with shellfish allergies.

5. _____ It is acceptable to palpate a puncture site again after cleaning as long as the PBT wears gloves.

6. _____ Isopropyl alcohol and tincture of iodine are the most common antiseptic agents for venipuncture to measure blood alcohol levels.

7. _____ When iodine is used as an antiseptic, it must later be removed from the skin with an alcohol prep pad.

8. _____ Chlorhexidine gluconate is often used to clean a site for a blood culture draw.

6. Identify techniques for proper needle placement and insertion

Short Answer

1. Describe the angle at which a needle should be held as it is inserted during venipuncture. Why is this important?

2. How should a PBT proceed if, after inserting the needle, blood does not flow? What action should be avoided and why?

3. Describe 4 things that can happen to prevent blood flow after a needle is inserted.

4. What should a PBT do if blood flow cannot be established?

7. Describe procedures for routine venipuncture

Fill in the Blank

1. Most venipuncture procedures are done in the _____ area of the arm with a straight _____ multisample needle and evacuated tubes.

Name: _____

2. Expired or damaged equipment must be properly _____.

3. A tourniquet cannot stay in place for more than _____ _____.

4. After the vein is punctured, the tourniquet is _____ as soon as blood flow begins.

5. Compared to butterfly needles, standard multisample needles are _____ to handle and pose _____ of a risk of accidental needle stick.

6. Before inserting the needle, tell the patient that she may feel brief _____ as the needle enters the skin.

7. The skin is punctured and the needle inserted into the selected vein in a(n) _____, _____ motion.

8. Most citrate and serum tubes require _____ inversions; most other tubes require _____.

9. After venipuncture, bleeding may take as long as _____ _____ to stop for patients on anticoagulant medications.

Multiple Choice

10. Why might a discard tube be used when drawing blood with a winged collection set?
    (A) Because the first blood drawn is not representative of the patient's blood overall
    (B) Because the air in the winged collection set tubing may interfere with proper filling of the collection tube
    (C) To ensure that the needle is properly in place within the vein
    (D) To have a backup supply of the patient's blood in case more tests are needed

11. When cleaning a venipuncture site the PBT should
    (A) Ask the patient their preferred level of pressure
    (B) Apply little to no pressure
    (C) Create gentle friction
    (D) Press down very firmly

12. How are inversions performed?
    (A) The collection tube is gently turned upside down and then right side up again.
    (B) The collection tube is shaken gently while being held upright, then shaken gently while being held upside down.
    (C) The collection tube is placed on a flat surface and spun gently.
    (D) The collection tube is shaken vigorously, then turned upside down and right side up again.

13. Which of the following is an acceptable way to make veins appear more prominently on the back of a patient's hand?
    (A) Ask the patient to hold her breath
    (B) Rub the patient's hand vigorously
    (C) Tighten the tourniquet
    (D) Ask the patient to form a fist

14. After cleaning a venipuncture site, what should the PBT do?
    (A) Insert the needle immediately
    (B) Fan the site until it is dry, then insert the needle
    (C) Count to 10, then insert the needle
    (D) Wait until the site air-dries, then insert the needle

15. When and where should a PBT label and initial the collection tubes and mark them with the time and date?
    (A) At a workstation at the beginning of the day
    (B) Before the blood draw is done, in front of the patient
    (C) After the blood draw is complete, in front of the patient
    (D) At a workstation at the end of the day

16. What should a PBT do if, at the point of inserting the needle, a patient says he does not consent to a blood draw?
    (A) Tell the patient it is too late to refuse
    (B) Tell the patient the general consent in his medical record applies and the draw must continue
    (C) Allow the patient to leave and document the refusal
    (D) Tell the patient he is making a serious mistake

8. Discuss adaptations to routine venipuncture for special populations and conditions

Matching
Match the following adaptations to the related population/condition. Letters may be used more than once.

1. ____ Ask a caregiver to help keep the patient still
2. ____ Draw blood on the nonoperative side
3. ____ Use a syringe and transfer device
4. ____ Position the patient in a reclined or supine position
5. ____ May need written permission from a provider for a blood draw
6. ____ Use smaller collection tubes (2 possible answers)
7. ____ Take special care with vein location, allowing the arm to dangle and/or using a warm pack
8. ____ Use a device that chills and/or vibrates above the puncture site
9. ____ Release the tourniquet and remove, sheath, and discard the needle immediately
10. ____ Use a longer needle

(A) Patients with small and/or fragile veins
(B) Pediatric patients
(C) Patients who are obese
(D) Patients who are prone to fainting
(E) A patient having a seizure or fainting
(F) Patients who have had mastectomies

Short Answer

11. When drawing blood from a patient with a cognitive impairment, where should the PBT keep supplies?

12. What should a PBT do if a patient says he feels faint?

13. List 3 examples of situations in which a PBT should not draw blood from an arm.

14. Describe how a PBT should respond to a patient who has a phobia related to needles or blood.

9. Identify guidelines for ensuring specimen integrity

Matching
For each of the following actions by a PBT, choose the letter that matches the type of error that may result. Letters may be used more than once.

1. ____ Mixing blood specimens with tube additives by shaking
2. ____ Not performing enough inversions
3. ____ Filling a tube about halfway to the fill line

Name: _____

4. _____ Telling a patient to pump her fist to help with vein selection

5. _____ Using a smaller needle than necessary

6. _____ Drawing multiple tubes without using correct order of draw

7. _____ Leaving a tourniquet on too long (2 possible answers)

8. _____ Labeling tubes before collection

9. _____ Pulling forcefully on a syringe plunger

10. _____ Drawing blood when a patient has just sat up from a supine position

11. _____ Transferring blood drawn with a syringe to a collection tube by puncturing the stopper with the collection needle

12. _____ Not trying to fill a tube completely/not trying a new tube when blood flow stops mid-collection

13. _____ Not asking a patient to confirm that identifying information on a collection tube label is correct

(A) Identification error

(B) Additive-related error

(C) Hemoconcentration

(D) Hemolysis

(E) Insufficient quantity

10. Describe special collections

True or False

1. _____ Chain of custody documentation is often required for blood culture tests.

2. _____ Glucose tolerance tests take longer than glucose challenge tests.

3. _____ Stoppers on blood culture collection bottles must be cleaned with alcohol swabs and allowed to dry before collection begins.

4. _____ In glucose tolerance testing, an initial specimen is drawn before the patient drinks the glucose beverage.

5. _____ Red-topped tubes are most commonly used for glucose testing.

6. _____ Ethanol is the intoxicating ingredient in alcoholic beverages.

7. _____ In some states a specimen for blood alcohol testing may be drawn even over the objection of the patient (i.e., without the patient's consent).

8. _____ Standard blood culture draws involve filling 4 culture bottles from a single venipuncture site.

9. _____ Avoiding transfers of specimens for blood cultures reduces the risk of contamination.

10. _____ Blood culture specimens may be collected in yellow-topped ACD tubes.

Short Answer

11. Use numbers 1–7 to correctly order the steps in collecting a blood culture specimen. (Note that there are steps on this page and the following page.) Assume the patient has already been correctly identified and the requisition checked.

_____ Clean the site with the second agent, following facility policy about time of contact with the skin. Allow it to air-dry completely.

_____ Collect the specimen in the anaerobic bottle.

_____ Gather supplies, including a winged collection set, 2 antiseptic agents, and blood culture bottles.

_____ Collect the specimen in the aerobic bottle.

_____ Clean the rubber stoppers on all collection bottles, each with a new alcohol prep pad. Allow them to dry.

____ After locating an appropriate vein, clean the site with the first antiseptic agent and allow it to air-dry completely.

____ Collect specimens for any other tests ordered, following correct order of draw.

12. Describe the difference between a glucose challenge test and a glucose tolerance test.

_____
_____
_____
_____
_____
_____
_____
_____
_____

13. Why may chain of custody documentation be required when testing for blood alcohol levels?

_____
_____
_____
_____

11. Discuss the processing and transportation of blood specimens

Matching
Use each letter only once.

1. ____ Centrifugation
2. ____ Aliquots
3. ____ Pipette
4. ____ Serum tubes
5. ____ Serum filter
6. ____ Heating block
7. ____ Ice slurry

(A) Mixture of crushed ice and water used to keep specimens cold

(B) Device inserted into a specimen tube to prevent the solid materials from mixing with the liquid portion

(C) Smaller amounts taken from a larger specimen for testing

(D) Rack designed to hold tubes upright at a specific temperature

(E) Spinning of samples to separate solid and liquid components

(F) Must be allowed to clot fully before centrifugation

(G) A narrow tube with a suction bulb; used to remove the liquid portion of a specimen

Multiple Choice

8. What does it mean to balance a centrifuge load?
    (A) To only centrifuge tubes with the same chemical additive
    (B) To only centrifuge tubes of the same size
    (C) To place tubes evenly within the centrifuge
    (D) To only centrifuge specimens 1 time

9. CLSI standards require centrifugation within _____ of collection, but some specimens may need to be centrifuged sooner.
    (A) 30 minutes
    (B) 1 hour
    (C) 2 hours
    (D) 1 day

10. Plasma or serum should be
    (A) Cloudy and milky
    (B) Tinted orange
    (C) Tinted deep yellow
    (D) Clear and straw-colored

Name: _____

11. When separating serum or plasma, how should a PBT remove the stopper from a specimen?
    (A) Using a special tool, if available, or carefully by hand
    (B) With a standard bottle opener
    (C) By popping it off with the thumb
    (D) By gently knocking it against the counter

12. Which of the following is an acceptable way to protect light-sensitive specimens?
    (A) By completing the draw in a darkened room
    (B) By using an amber or foil-wrapped collection tube
    (C) By asking the patient to hold the tube in cupped hands to block light
    (D) By placing the tube in a centrifuge immediately after collection and closing the lid

13. A lipemic specimen is most likely in which of the following cases?
    (A) The patient has been fasting.
    (B) The patient is jaundiced.
    (C) The collection tube was shaken to mix, rather than being inverted gently.
    (D) The patient had a breakfast of bacon and eggs.

Short Answer

14. List 3 common ways specimens are transported from where they are drawn to where there are tested.

    _____
    _____
    _____
    _____

15. List at least 1 analyte that must be protected from light. Describe how specimens are protected from light.

    _____
    _____
    _____

16. List at least 1 analyte that must be kept cold. Describe how specimens are kept cold.

    _____
    _____
    _____
    _____

17. List at least 1 analyte that must be kept at body temperature. Describe how specimens are kept warm.

    _____
    _____
    _____
    _____

18. What steps should a PBT follow after they have finished processing and preparing specimens for transport?

    _____
    _____
    _____
    _____
    _____
    _____
    _____
    _____

Please do not copy our workbook. Report violations to legal@hartmanonline.com.

Name: _____

Name: _____

10

Collecting Blood Specimens by Capillary (Dermal) Puncture

1. List the most common situations in which capillary puncture is required

Short Answer
Place a check mark (✓) next to descriptions of patients who may need to have blood specimens taken by capillary puncture rather than venipuncture.

1. ____ Patients with burned or heavily scarred arms
2. ____ Patients who are between the ages of 2 and 12
3. ____ Patients who are dehydrated
4. ____ Patients whose veins are very fragile or damaged
5. ____ Patients whose veins are difficult to see
6. ____ Patients whose veins must be used only for treatments such as chemotherapy
7. ____ Patients who have bruises on their hands

Short Answer

8. What are 2 types of blood tests that cannot be performed on a capillary specimen?

   _____
   _____

9. Why is a capillary specimen better than a venous specimen for testing blood gases?

   _____
   _____
   _____

10. Capillary puncture is used to collect specimens from small infants. What is one reason for this?

    _____
    _____
    _____
    _____

11. What causes iatrogenic anemia?

    _____
    _____
    _____
    _____

12. Why should the type of specimen taken (e.g., capillary) always be documented?

    _____
    _____
    _____
    _____

13. Blood volume in infants (in mL) may be estimated to be 80 × the infant's weight (in kg). To prevent iatrogenic anemia, no more than 5% of a patient's blood volume should be drawn in 30 days. What is the maximum amount of blood that can be drawn in a one-month period from an infant who weighs 2.5 kg?

    _____

2. Discuss the selection of an appropriate site for capillary puncture

True or False

1. ____ Capillary specimens are usually collected from the index finger.

2. ____ The earlobe is considered an appropriate site if another site is difficult to find.

3. ____ The fact that the bone is close to the tip of the smallest finger (pinky or fifth finger) makes it a poor choice for capillary collection.

4. ____ Because there is a pulse point in the thumb, it is a good choice for capillary collection.

5. ____ If a patient is undergoing capillary blood testing frequently, the sites should be rotated.

6. ____ A finger stick should not be performed on an infant who weighs less than 10 kilograms.

7. ____ The very tip of the finger should be avoided when performing capillary puncture.

8. ____ The *calcaneus* is the part of an infant's foot with the best blood flow.

9. ____ The medial and lateral plantar surfaces of the heel are both acceptable areas for heel stick.

10. ____ When selecting a site for a heelstick collection, the PBT must avoid sites close to bone due to the risk of osteomyelitis.

Short Answer
Read the following and mark whether or not they are examples of situations that could cause a problem for capillary collection. Write P for potential problems and N for situations that are not likely to cause problems.

11. ____ The patient has been drinking water steadily all morning.

12. ____ The patient feels very cold and the beds of his fingernails are blue.

13. ____ The patient had a mastectomy on her right side.

14. ____ The patient's hands and arms are covered in burn scars.

3. Describe the proper cleaning of a capillary puncture site

Multiple Choice

1. Which antiseptic should not be used before capillary puncture due to possible interference with analytes?
   (A) Chlorhexidine gluconate
   (B) Povidone-iodine
   (C) 70% isopropyl alcohol
   (D) Sodium hypochlorite

2. What should a PBT do if a patient's hands are visibly dirty?
   (A) Ask the patient to come back another day
   (B) Use at least 2 alcohol prep pads to clean the fingerstick site
   (C) Use 2 different antiseptics (e.g., chlorhexidine gluconate and an alcohol prep pad)
   (D) Ask the patient to wash their hands

3. What must happen after an antiseptic is used on a capillary puncture site?
   (A) The patient's skin must look flushed from the friction.
   (B) The patient must wash their hands.
   (C) The antiseptic must be allowed to dry completely.
   (D) The skin must be wiped dry with a gauze pad.

4. Friction must be used when cleaning a puncture site, but special care must be taken with the skin of patients who
   (A) Are infants or elderly people
   (B) Have phobias about blood draws
   (C) Have very deep fingerprint lines
   (D) Have blood taken by capillary puncture frequently

4. Identify techniques for proper preparation and puncture of the skin

True or False

1. ____ A lancet blade should be placed in line with a patient's fingerprint lines.

Name: _____

2. ____ The same type of lancet is used for all capillary puncture procedures.

3. ____ Microcollection tubes, capillary tubes, and filter paper are all possible collection devices for capillary puncture.

4. ____ Heelstick procedures are usually performed using 0.85 mm or 1.0 mm blade-style lancets.

5. ____ When collecting a capillary specimen from an adult, the size of lancet used may depend on the amount of blood that must be collected.

6. ____ A button-activated lancet should be pressed firmly into a patient's skin before the button is pressed.

7. ____ Light-blocking amber microcollection tubes may be used when bilirubin testing is performed on infants.

Short Answer

8. List items that should be close by before the PBT punctures a patient's skin to collect a capillary specimen.

_____
_____
_____
_____
_____

9. What is usually done with the first drop of blood during capillary collection? List 2 reasons for doing this.

_____
_____
_____
_____
_____

10. List 2 effects of warming a capillary puncture site before collecting a specimen. List 2 ways to warm a capillary puncture site.

_____
_____
_____
_____
_____
_____
_____

5. Describe procedures for routine capillary puncture in the finger and the heel

Multiple Choice

1. When should a specimen be collected by capillary puncture?
   (A) When it is ordered to be collected by capillary puncture
   (B) When a phlebotomy technician cannot find an acceptable vein for venipuncture
   (C) When the patient requests it
   (D) When the patient has fragile veins

2. A 2-mm lancet is most likely to be used for
   (A) An infant
   (B) A toddler
   (C) A school-aged child
   (D) An adult

3. Which type of tube would be filled first when taking a capillary specimen?
   (A) Citrate tube
   (B) Tube with no additive
   (C) EDTA tube
   (D) Clot activator tube

4. How should a 3-year-old child be positioned for capillary puncture?
   (A) In a trusted adult's lap
   (B) In the lap of another healthcare worker
   (C) Supine on an examination table
   (D) On a booster seat

Fill in the Blank

5. Always select a new finger if a(n) _____ _____ is required.

6. Check equipment carefully for _____ and, as applicable, for _____ dates. Discard _____ or faulty equipment.

7. Ensure there is no _____ or _____ in the patient's mouth.

8. Ask the patient to extend their hands, _____ _____ for a visual inspection.

9. Once a lancet is prepared, it must be used _____ or discarded. If it is put down, it is considered to be _____.

10. After use, a lancet is discarded in a(n) _____ _____.

11. During specimen collection, do not _____ or _____ the patient's finger.

12. Do not touch the _____ to the patient's skin.

13. Tubes must be labeled _____ _____ _____ the patient.

14. Before allowing a patient to leave, the PBT should check to make sure the patient is no longer _____.

Matching
Use each letter only once.

15. _____ Heel stick
16. _____ Bilirubin
17. _____ Premature infants
18. _____ Adhesive bandages
19. _____ Nursing and swaddling
20. _____ Finger stick
21. _____ Antiseptics

(A) May reduce pain experienced during capillary puncture

(B) Often tested in infants

(C) May irritate infant skin; follow facility policy for use

(D) Require use of a smaller lancet

(E) Should not be used on infants

(F) Must be used when collecting capillary specimens from small infants

(G) May be used on infants at least 6 months old and weighing at least 10 kg

6. Identify guidelines for ensuring the integrity of capillary puncture specimens

Short Answer

1. During a capillary collection, what action should be avoided? How can a PBT best promote blood flow while avoiding this action?

   _____
   _____
   _____
   _____
   _____

2. How high should microcollection tubes be filled?

   _____
   _____

3. Why is it important for a phlebotomy technician to work quickly to collect a specimen after a capillary puncture is performed?

   _____
   _____
   _____

4. Why should capillary specimens not be collected from sites where a patient is experiencing edema?

   _____
   _____
   _____

Name: _____

5. What type of damage may be caused to a specimen if a patient's finger or heel is squeezed excessively?

_____

6. What is one sign a phlebotomist should observe for that may indicate poor circulation?

_____
_____

7. Describe special capillary puncture collections

Multiple Choice

1. Blood gases are usually tested using
   (A) Capillary blood
   (B) Arterial blood
   (C) Venous blood
   (D) Breath exhaled from the lungs

2. What comes first in the capillary puncture order of draw if blood gases are being tested?
   (A) The blood gas specimen
   (B) EDTA tubes
   (C) Non-additive tubes
   (D) Heparin tubes

3. As much as possible, a capillary specimen for blood gas testing should not come into contact with
   (A) The lancet
   (B) The collection device
   (C) Room air
   (D) The lid or seal on the collection device

4. What is the name of the small piece of metal used to mix a blood gas specimen?
   (A) A flea
   (B) A bug
   (C) A bit
   (D) A flange

5. Which of the following is an illness screened for in all states that require infant metabolic screening?
   (A) Phenylketonuria (PKU)
   (B) Jaundice
   (C) Down syndrome
   (D) Measles

6. When collecting a specimen for newborn metabolic screening, what should the completed collection card look like?
   (A) Each circle should have a single, small drop of blood in the center, with clean paper around the edges.
   (B) The blood should be centered in each circle, but should extend past the lines so that it touches the drop in the next circle.
   (C) Each circle should be fully covered and soaked through, with the blood visible on both the front and the back of the paper.
   (D) The blood should be dripped onto the back of the paper so that it is just visible inside the circles on the front.

True or False

7. _____ A blood smear may be used to test for bloodborne parasites.

8. _____ A blood smear may be used to observe for changes or problems with a patient's blood cells.

9. _____ To create a blood smear, a spreader is placed at a 90-degree angle and pulled across a drop of blood on a microscope slide.

10. _____ A second clean, unused microscope slide may be used in place of a spreader if necessary.

11. _____ Blood for a blood smear is collected in a heparinized capillary tube.

12. _____ The edge of a blood smear should look like a thick, solid line.

13. _____ Blood smears must be transported for testing while they are still wet.

8. Describe guidelines for performing point-of-care tests on capillary blood

Short Answer

1. List 4 common point-of-care tests performed on capillary blood.

_____
_____

2. How is point-of-care blood testing usually performed?

3. What may a phlebotomy technician need to do with a point-of-care testing device before using it to test a patient's blood?

4. In what situation(s) might a PBT need to discard unused test strips?

5. After point-of-care testing, a patient asks a PBT what the result is and what it means. How should the PBT respond?

6. What is a critical value? Why should PBTs know critical values for any point-of-care tests they perform?

7. What will a PBT likely be asked to do when a point-of-care test produces a result in the critical value range?

8. What must be done with a point-of-care testing device after every use (if it is not used by a single patient)?

9. Where should used test strips be discarded?

11

Nonblood Specimens

1. Identify nonblood specimens collected for laboratory testing

Fill in the Blank

1. After blood, _____ is the most commonly tested type of specimen.

2. Swabs are often used to collect specimens to determine whether _____ or other _____ are present.

3. Swabs may also be used to collect _____ for analysis, as in DNA testing.

4. In some cases specimens are _____, or drawn out by suction, usually through a(n) _____ inserted in the patient's body.

5. Only _____ or other specially trained healthcare professionals collect specimens by needle aspiration.

Matching
Use each letter only once.

6. _____ Pericardial fluid
7. _____ Amniotic fluid
8. _____ Bone marrow
9. _____ Peritoneal fluid
10. _____ Synovial fluid
11. _____ Pleural fluid
12. _____ Cerebrospinal fluid

(A) Fluid from the area around the joints
(B) Fluid from the sac surrounding a fetus
(C) Fluid from the abdominal cavity
(D) Fluid from the area surrounding the brain and spinal column
(E) Fluid from the lining of the heart
(F) Tissue from the center of the bones
(G) Fluid from the lining of the lungs

2. Describe types of urine specimens and demonstrate how to collect a clean-catch urine specimen

Short Answer

1. What is the difference between a routine urine specimen and a clean-catch urine specimen?

2. When does a first void urine specimen need to be collected?

3. What type of urine test may be ordered when a patient has repeated or severe UTIs?

4. What methods may be used to collect a urine specimen from a patient who is unable to urinate normally? What role may the PBT have related to these specimens?

_____
_____
_____
_____

5. How may a urine specimen be collected from a child who still wears diapers?

_____
_____
_____

6. What is the usual time frame for testing urine specimens after collection?

_____
_____

True or False

7. _____ A postprandial urine specimen is collected immediately after a patient has eaten a meal.

8. _____ Gloves should always be worn when handling urine specimens.

9. _____ The lid is the best place to put a label on a urine specimen container.

10. _____ Routine urine specimens are collected in sterile containers.

11. _____ Patients should be instructed to fill urine specimen containers at least half full.

12. _____ When collecting a clean-catch (midstream) specimen, the patient should wash hands before starting the collection procedure.

13. _____ Females should clean the labia and the urethral opening before providing a clean-catch urine specimen.

14. _____ Males do not need to clean the genital area before providing a clean-catch urine specimen.

15. _____ Patients giving specimens for drug testing must generally be identified by photo ID.

16. _____ Water is usually turned off in the bathroom where a urine specimen is being collected for drug testing.

17. _____ The temperature of urine specimens for drug testing must be checked within half an hour of voiding.

18. _____ Creating a *split specimen* involves asking a patient to void into 2 separate cups over the course of an hour.

19. _____ Patients must seal and initial their own specimens when urine is collected for drug testing.

20. _____ Patients should not be allowed to wear coats or bulky clothing into the bathroom when providing a urine specimen for drug testing.

Multiple Choice

21. What is one reason PBTs should warn patients to avoid splashing when pouring urine into a 24-hour urine specimen container?
    (A) Because the containers sometimes have caustic chemical additives inside
    (B) Because it will reduce the amount of urine available to test
    (C) Because it will cause test results to be inaccurate
    (D) Because splashing urine may make the label difficult to read

22. What happens to the first urine a patient voids on the morning a 24-hour urine collection begins?
    (A) It is collected in a separate specimen cup and turned in along with the larger container.
    (B) It is voided directly into the toilet and not collected.
    (C) It is held in a separate container and added only if the volume of urine after 24 hours is not high enough.
    (D) It is added to the large collection container as the first urine of the 24-hour collection.

Name: _____

23. When preparing a patient for a 24-hour collection, what equipment is often sent home with the patient?
    (A) Test tubes holding chemical agents the patient must add to the specimen
    (B) A collection bag with adhesive that is fitted over the genitals
    (C) Wipes for cleaning the genital area before each void
    (D) A hat for the toilet and/or a urinal

24. A urine specific gravity test
    (A) Checks for adequate oxygen levels
    (B) Indicates the specific type of urinary incontinence a patient is experiencing
    (C) Counts the amount of blood cells in urine
    (D) Shows how the density of urine compares to the density of water

25. The presence of glucose or ketones in urine may be a sign of
    (A) High blood pressure
    (B) Thyroid disorder
    (C) Anemia
    (D) Diabetes

26. A double-voided urine specimen may be used to test for
    (A) Glucose
    (B) Sweat
    (C) Sputum
    (D) Nitrites

27. One type of reagent (dip) strip test measures how acidic or alkaline urine is; it measures the _____.
    (A) Food
    (B) pH level
    (C) Illegal drugs
    (D) Fat

28. Occult blood in urine is
    (A) A normal change of aging
    (B) Easily seen
    (C) Hidden
    (D) A sign of anemia

3. Describe tests performed on stool and instructions for handling a stool specimen

Short Answer

1. What are 4 things a stool sample may be tested for?

   _____
   _____
   _____
   _____

2. Briefly describe the 2 types of fecal occult blood testing.

   _____
   _____
   _____
   _____
   _____
   _____
   _____
   _____
   _____
   _____
   _____
   _____

3. List 4 items that patients are asked not to consume before and during fecal guaiac testing.

   _____
   _____
   _____
   _____
   _____
   _____

4. What 3 things should patients be asked not to include in a stool sample?

_____

_____

_____

4. Demonstrate how to obtain a throat culture and discuss other swabbing procedures

Fill in the Blank

1. The swabbing procedure most likely to be performed by a phlebotomy technician is a(n) _____ _____.

2. Allow children to sit in a(n) _____ _____ during a swabbing procedure if they wish to do so.

3. When swabbing the throat do not touch the patient's _____. This can cause a(n) _____ reflex.

4. Some swabs, once a specimen has been collected, are stored in a vial with a(n) _____, or small container of liquid, that must be crushed.

5. Gently supporting the back of the patient's _____ during the procedure can help steady him until the procedure is over.

Matching
Use each letter only once.

6. ____ Nasopharyngeal aspirate

7. ____ Nasal swab

8. ____ Throat culture

9. ____ Buccal swab

10. ____ Nasopharyngeal swab

(A) Involves introducing sterile saline solution into the nasal cavity

(B) Involves taking cells from the inside of the patient's cheek (e.g., for DNA analysis)

(C) Involves the nostrils

(D) Often used to test for influenza

(E) Used to test for strep throat

5. Describe guidelines for the collection and handling of other nonblood specimens

Multiple Choice

1. What type of bacteria is tested for when a breath test is performed?
   (A) *Streptococcus pyogenes*
   (B) *Clostridioides difficile*
   (C) Methicillin-resistant *Streptococcus aureus*
   (D) *Helicobacter pylori*

2. Semen specimens must be kept close to this temperature:
   (A) Freezing temperature
   (B) Body temperature
   (C) Room temperature
   (D) Boiling temperature

3. How quickly must a patient deliver a semen specimen to the laboratory?
   (A) Within 15 minutes
   (B) Within 30 minutes
   (C) Within 1 hour
   (D) Within 24 hours

4. When are sputum specimens most easily collected?
   (A) First thing in the morning
   (B) After the patient has exercised
   (C) After the patient has eaten a full meal
   (D) Right before bed

5. What PPE should a phlebotomy technician wear while collecting a sputum specimen?
   (A) Gloves
   (B) Gloves and a gown
   (C) Gloves and a surgical mask
   (D) Gloves and an N95 respirator

6. What must be included if a hair specimen will be tested for DNA?
   (A) The root of the hair
   (B) The tip of the hair
   (C) Any part of the hair that is not artificially colored
   (D) The middle of the hair shaft

Name: _____

7. Which of the following might be tested in saliva?
   (A) Hormone levels
   (B) Fungus
   (C) Stomach acid
   (D) Blood alcohol

8. In addition to collecting and handling specimens according to quality standards, what is the job of the phlebotomy technician?
   (A) To answer all patient questions
   (B) To explain to the patient the purpose of tests and the meaning of results
   (C) To provide friendly, professional customer service to the patient
   (D) To manage the workflow of a laboratory

Nonblood Specimens

Name: _____

Name: _____

Procedure Checklists

	Washing hands (hand hygiene)	yes	no
1.	Turns on the water at the sink. Keeps clothes dry and does not let clothing touch the outside portion of the sink or counter.		
2.	Wets hands and wrists thoroughly.		
3.	Applies soap to hands.		
4.	Keeps hands lower than elbows and fingertips down. Rubs hands together and fingers between each other to create a lather. Lathers all surfaces of wrists, hands, and fingers, using friction for at least 20 seconds.		
5.	Cleans fingernails by rubbing them in the palm of other hand.		
6.	Keeps hands lower than elbows and fingertips down. Rinses all surfaces of wrists and hands. Runs water down from wrists to fingertips. Does not run water over unwashed arms down to clean hands.		
7.	Uses a clean, dry paper towel to dry all surfaces of fingers, hands, and wrists, starting at the fingertips. Does not wipe the towel on unwashed forearms and then wipe clean hands. Discards the towel in the waste container without touching the container. Starts over if hands touch the sink or wastebasket.		
8.	Uses a clean, dry paper towel to turn off the faucet. Discards the towel in the waste container. Does not contaminate hands by touching the surface of the sink or faucet.		

_____   _____
Date Reviewed   Instructor Signature

_____   _____
Date Performed   Instructor Signature

Name: _____

Putting on (donning) and removing (doffing) a gown		yes	no
1.	Washes hands.		
2.	Opens the gown. Allows the gown to open/unfold without shaking or touching it to the floor. Faces the back opening of the gown and places an arm through each sleeve.		
3.	Fastens the neck opening.		
4.	Reaches behind and pulls the gown until it completely covers clothing. Secures the gown at waist.		
5.	Puts on gloves after putting on the gown with cuffs of the gloves overlapping the cuffs of the gown.		
6.	When removing the gown, first removes and discards gloves properly, then unfastens the gown at the waist and neck. Removes the gown without touching the outside of the gown. Rolls the dirty side in, holding the gown away from the body. Discards the gown properly and washes hands.		

_____ _____
Date Reviewed   Instructor Signature

_____ _____
Date Performed   Instructor Signature

Name: _____

Putting on (donning) a mask and goggles			
		yes	no
1.	Washes hands.		
2.	Picks up the mask by the top strings or the elastic strap. Does not touch the mask where it touches the face.		
3.	Pulls the elastic strap over the head, or if the mask has strings, ties the top strings first, then the bottom strings.		
4.	Pinches the metal strip at the top of the mask (if part of the mask) tightly around the nose and fits the mask snugly around the face and below the chin.		
5.	Places the goggles over eyes or eyeglasses. Uses the headband or earpieces to secure them to the head. Makes sure they are on snugly.		
6.	Puts on gloves after putting on the mask and goggles.		

_____ _____
Date Reviewed   Instructor Signature

_____ _____
Date Performed   Instructor Signature

Name: _____

	Putting on (donning) gloves	yes	no
1.	Washes hands.		
2.	Slides 1 glove on.		
3.	Using the gloved hand, slides the other hand into the second glove.		
4.	Interlaces fingers to smooth out folds and create a comfortable fit.		
5.	Carefully checks for tears, holes, or discolored spots, replacing gloves if needed.		
6.	Adjusts the gloves until they are pulled up over the wrist and fit correctly. If wearing a gown, pulls the cuffs of the gloves over the sleeves of the gown.		

_____ _____
Date Reviewed   Instructor Signature

_____ _____
Date Performed   Instructor Signature

Name: _____

Removing (doffing) gloves		yes	no
1.	Touches only the outside of 1 glove. With 1 gloved hand, grasps the other glove at the palm and pulls the glove off.		
2.	With the fingertips of the gloved hand, holds the removed glove. Slips 2 fingers of the ungloved hand underneath the cuff of the remaining glove at the wrist. Does not touch any part of the outside of the glove.		
3.	Pulls down, turning the glove inside out and over the first glove as it is removed.		
4.	Holds 1 glove from its clean inner side with the other glove inside it.		
5.	Drops both gloves into the proper container.		
6.	Washes hands.		

_____   _____
Date Reviewed   Instructor Signature

_____   _____
Date Performed   Instructor Signature

Name: _____

Donning a full set of PPE		yes	no
1.	Washes hands.		
2.	Puts on gown.		
3.	Puts on mask and respirator.		
4.	Puts on goggles or face shield.		
5.	Puts on gloves.		

_____ _____
Date Reviewed   Instructor Signature

_____ _____
Date Performed   Instructor Signature

Name: _____

Doffing a full set of PPE			
		yes	no
1.	Removes and discards gloves.		
2.	Removes and discards goggles and face shield.		
3.	Removes and discards gown.		
4.	Removes and discards mask.		
5.	Washes hands.		

_____   _____
Date Reviewed   Instructor Signature

_____   _____
Date Performed   Instructor Signature

Name: _____

	Performing routine venipuncture with multisample needle and evacuated tube(s)	yes	no
1.	Greets the patient. Identifies self by name and title.		
2.	Identifies the patient using 2 unique identifiers.		
3.	Explains the procedure to the patient. Ensures consent.		
4.	Gathers required equipment.		
5.	Washes (or sanitizes) hands. Dons gloves and other PPE as required.		
6.	Asks the patient to extend arms for a visual inspection. Chooses an arm based on the appearance of the veins and the patient's input.		
7.	Applies the tourniquet to the selected arm, 3–4 inches above the bend in the elbow. Asks the patient to make (but not pump) a fist.		
8.	With a gloved index finger, palpates the arm to locate an acceptable vein, with a preference for the median veins. If an acceptable site is not found, removes the tourniquet and applies it to the other arm.		
9.	When a suitable site is located, releases the tourniquet and cleans the site thoroughly. Applies friction with the alcohol pad (or other antiseptic agent).		
10.	Allows the alcohol to dry fully. Does not blow on, fan, or wipe the skin to speed drying. Assembles the needle and holder.		
11.	Reapplies the tourniquet.		
12.	Anchors the vein. Uses the thumb to apply pressure and pulls the skin toward the wrist an inch or 2 below the venipuncture site. Does not place an anchoring finger above the venipuncture site.		
13.	In a single, fluid motion, inserts the needle into the skin to puncture the selected vein at an angle of less than 30 degrees.		
14.	Inserts the first collection tube. As soon as blood flow is established, releases the tourniquet. Allows the tube to fill completely.		
15.	If multiple tubes are required, replaces the first filled tube with the next tube according to proper order of draw. Continues until all necessary tubes are filled.		
16.	Places a piece of gauze, folded into quarters, over the needle.		
17.	Withdraws the needle from the patient's arm, engaging the safety device. Disposes of the needle and holder in an appropriate sharps receptacle. Maintains pressure on the gauze, asking the patient to assist as able. Does not allow the patient to bend arm up.		
18.	Mixes tubes appropriately, gently turning the tube upside down and then right side up again.		
19.	Labels the tubes in front of the patient, initialing and noting the time and date of collection. Asks the patient to confirm that the identifying information on the label is correct. Places the specimens and the requisition or any required paperwork in the appropriate transport bag or container. Properly discards any waste.		
20.	Checks to make sure that the patient is no longer bleeding.		
21.	Places a bandage over the gauze on the patient's arm. Advises the patient to leave the bandage in place for the next 15 minutes.		
22.	Observes the patient for any signs of dizziness or discomfort.		
23.	Thanks the patient.		
24.	Removes gloves and washes hands.		
25.	Documents the procedure according to facility policy.		

_____   _____
Date Reviewed   Instructor Signature

_____   _____
Date Performed   Instructor Signature

Name: _____

Performing venipuncture in the hand with winged collection system and evacuated tube(s)

		yes	no
1.	Greets the patient. Identifies self by name and title.		
2.	Identifies the patient using 2 unique identifiers.		
3.	Explains the procedure to the patient. Ensures consent.		
4.	Gathers required equipment.		
5.	Washes (or sanitizes) hands. Dons gloves and other PPE as required.		
6.	Asks the patient to extend hands, palms down, for a visual inspection. Chooses a hand based on the appearance of the veins and the patient's input.		
7.	Applies the tourniquet to the forearm above the selected hand, 3–4 inches above the intended puncture site. Asks the patient to make (but not pump) a fist.		
8.	With a gloved index finger, palpates the vein and determines the best site for puncture. If an acceptable site is not found, removes the tourniquet and applies it to the other forearm.		
9.	When a suitable site is located, releases the tourniquet and cleans the site thoroughly. Applies friction with the alcohol pad (or other antiseptic agent).		
10.	Allows the alcohol to dry fully. Does not blow on, fan, or wipe the skin to speed drying. Prepares the winged collection set and holder.		
11.	Reapplies the tourniquet.		
12.	Anchors the vein. Uses the thumb to apply pressure and pulls the skin toward the wrist an inch or 2 below the venipuncture site. Does not place an anchoring finger above the venipuncture site.		
13.	In a single, fluid motion, inserts the needle into the skin to puncture the selected vein at an angle of less than 30 degrees. Releases tourniquet after accessing the vein.		
14.	Secures the needle of a winged collection set throughout the draw, following CLSI standards.		
15.	If a discard tube is needed, inserts it first, then removes and discards it in the sharps container as soon as blood enters it. Inserts the first collection tube. Allows it to fill completely.		
16.	If multiple tubes are required, replaces the first filled tube with the next tube according to proper order of draw. Continues until all necessary tubes are filled.		
17.	Places a piece of gauze, folded into quarters, over the needle.		
18.	Withdraws the needle from the patient's hand, engaging the safety device. Discards the needle, tubing, and holder in an appropriate sharps receptacle. Maintains pressure on the gauze, asking the patient to assist as able.		
19.	Mixes tubes appropriately, gently turning the tube upside down and then right side up again.		
20.	Labels the tubes in front of the patient, initialing and noting the time and date of collection. Asks the patient to confirm that the identifying information on the label is correct. Places the specimens and the requisition or any required paperwork in the appropriate transport bag or container. Properly discards any waste.		
21.	Checks to make sure that the patient is no longer bleeding.		
22.	Places a bandage over the gauze on the patient's hand. Advises the patient to leave the bandage in place for the next 15 minutes.		

23.	Observes the patient for any signs of dizziness or discomfort.		
24.	Thanks the patient.		
25.	Removes gloves and washes hands.		
26.	Documents the procedure according to facility policy.		

_____   _____
Date Reviewed   Instructor Signature

_____   _____
Date Performed   Instructor Signature

Name: _____

Collecting a blood specimen using a syringe and transfer device

		yes	no
1.	Greets the patient. Identifies self by name and title.		
2.	Identifies the patient using 2 unique identifiers.		
3.	Explains the procedure to the patient. Ensures consent.		
4.	Gathers required equipment.		
5.	Washes (or sanitizes) hands. Dons gloves and other PPE as required.		
6.	Asks the patient to extend arms or hands, palms down, for a visual inspection. Chooses an arm or hand based on the appearance of the veins and the patient's input.		
7.	Applies the tourniquet 3–4 inches above the selected area. Asks the patient to make (but not pump) a fist.		
8.	With a gloved index finger, palpates the vein and determines the best site for puncture. If an acceptable site is not found, removes the tourniquet and applies it to the other arm.		
9.	When a suitable site is located, releases the tourniquet and cleans the site thoroughly. Applies friction with the alcohol pad (or other antiseptic agent).		
10.	Allows the alcohol to dry fully. Does not blow on, fan, or wipe the skin to speed drying. Assembles the needle and syringe.		
11.	Prepares the syringe for use.		
12.	Reapplies the tourniquet.		
13.	Anchors the vein. Uses the thumb to apply pressure and pulls the skin toward self an inch or 2 below the venipuncture site. Does not place an anchoring finger above the venipuncture site.		
14.	In a single, fluid motion, inserts the needle into the skin to puncture the selected vein at an angle of less than 30 degrees. Releases the tourniquet after accessing the vein.		
15.	Secures the needle of a winged collection set throughout the draw, following CLSI standards.		
16.	Pulls back gently and steadily on the syringe plunger until the necessary volume of blood is collected.		
17.	Places a piece of gauze, folded into quarters, over the needle.		
18.	Withdraws the needle from the patient's body, engaging the safety device. Maintains pressure on the gauze, asking the patient to assist as able.		
19.	Removes flexible tubing from the syringe and places the needle and tubing in a sharps disposal container.		
20.	Immediately screws the syringe onto the syringe transfer device.		
21.	Inserts appropriate collection tube(s), according to order of draw. Does not press on the syringe plunger as the blood transfers, allowing the vacuum in the tube to draw the blood in to the required level.		
22.	Disposes of the syringe and transfer device in the sharps container.		
23.	Mixes tubes appropriately, gently turning the tube upside down and then right side up again.		
24.	Labels the tubes in front of the patient, initialing and noting the time and date of collection. Asks the patient to confirm that the identifying information on the label is correct. Places the specimens and the requisition or any required paperwork in the appropriate transport bag or container. Properly discards any waste.		

25.	Checks to make sure that the patient is no longer bleeding.		
26.	Places a bandage over the gauze on the patient's hand. Advises the patient to leave the bandage in place for the next 15 minutes.		
27.	Observes the patient for any signs of dizziness or discomfort.		
28.	Thanks the patient.		
29.	Removes gloves and washes hands.		
30.	Documents the procedure according to facility policy.		

_____ _____
Date Reviewed Instructor Signature

_____ _____
Date Performed Instructor Signature

Name: _____

Performing routine capillary puncture by finger stick			
		yes	no
1.	Greets the patient. Identifies self by name and title.		
2.	Identifies the patient using 2 unique identifiers.		
3.	Explains the procedure to the patient. Ensures consent.		
4.	Gathers required equipment.		
5.	Washes (or sanitizes) hands. Dons gloves and other PPE as required.		
6.	Asks the patient to extend hands, palms up, for a visual inspection. Chooses a puncture site free of bruising, rashes, broken skin (including recent capillary puncture), swelling, or cyanosis.		
7.	Warms the site if required.		
8.	Cleans the selected puncture site thoroughly, creating gentle friction. Allows the site to dry fully.		
9.	Prepares the selected lancet and collection devices for use.		
10.	Presses the lancet gently against the patient's skin at the selected puncture site and activates the lancet to puncture the skin.		
11.	Discards the used lancet in an appropriate sharps receptacle.		
12.	Uses a gauze square to wipe away the first drop of blood if required.		
13.	Collects the patient's blood in the required container(s). Applies gentle pressure. Does not squeeze or "milk" the finger. Gently applies and then releases pressure to facilitate blood flow. Does not touch the spout or any part of the collection device to the patient's skin. Allows the blood to drip into the tube, creating a channel down the side of the collection tube. Gently taps the collection tube as the blood enters to help mix the specimen with the anticoagulant.		
14.	Continues to hold the patient's finger and the collection device in place until the container is filled to the appropriate level. After filling, caps/seals the specimens appropriately and mixes them promptly.		
15.	After all required containers are filled, places gauze over the puncture site and applies pressure, allowing patient to assist as able.		
16.	Labels the tube(s) in front of the patient, initialing and noting the time and date of collection. Asks the patient to confirm that the identifying information on the label is correct. Places the specimens and the requisition or any required paperwork in the appropriate transport bag or container. Properly discards any waste.		
17.	Checks to make sure that the patient is no longer bleeding.		
18.	Places a bandage over the puncture site if the patient is over 2 years old. Advises the patient to leave the bandage in place for the next 15 minutes.		
19.	Observes the patient for any signs of dizziness or discomfort. Does not allow the patient to stand if she seems unsteady or says that she feels faint.		
20.	Thanks the patient.		
21.	Removes gloves and washes hands.		
22.	Documents the procedure according to facility policy.		

_____   _____
Date Reviewed   Instructor Signature

_____   _____
Date Performed   Instructor Signature

Name: _____

Performing routine capillary puncture by heel stick		
	yes	no
1.	Greets the patient's parent(s) or guardian(s). Identifies self by name and title.		
2.	Identifies the patient using 2 unique identifiers.		
3.	Explains the procedure to the parent/guardian. Ensures consent.		
4.	Gathers required equipment.		
5.	Washes (or sanitizes) hands. Dons gloves and other PPE as required.		
6.	If parent wishes to hold the baby during the procedure, places the baby in the parent's arms.		
7.	Warms the site for up to 5 minutes using a warm, damp cloth or a commercial warming pack.		
8.	Cleans the selected puncture site (medial or lateral plantar surface of either heel) thoroughly with the antiseptic pad, creating gentle friction. Allows the site to dry fully.		
9.	Prepares the lancet and collection devices for use.		
10.	Presses the lancet gently against the patient's skin at the selected puncture site and activates the lancet to puncture the skin.		
11.	Discards the used lancet in an appropriate sharps receptacle.		
12.	Uses a gauze square to wipe away the first drop of blood if the ordered test does not indicate otherwise.		
13.	Collects the patient's blood in the required container(s). Alternately applies and releases gentle pressure to the sides of the baby's heel. Does not touch the spout or any part of the collection device to the infant's skin. Allows the blood to drip into the tube and create a channel down the side of the collection tube. Gently taps the collection tube as the blood enters.		
14.	Continues to hold the baby's heel and the collection device in place until the container is filled to the appropriate level. After filling, caps/seals the specimens appropriately and mixes them promptly.		
15.	After all required containers are filled, places gauze over the puncture site and applies pressure.		
16.	When the puncture site is no longer bleeding, bandages the heel according to facility policy (does not use adhesive bandages).		
17.	Labels the tube(s) in front of the patient's parent(s) or guardian(s), initialing and noting the time and date of collection. Confirms that the identifying information on the label is correct. Places the specimens and the requisition or any required paperwork in the appropriate transport bag or container. Properly discards any waste.		
18.	Thanks the patient's parent or guardian.		
19.	Removes gloves and washes hands.		
20.	Documents the procedure according to facility policy.		

_____ _____
Date Reviewed   Instructor Signature

_____ _____
Date Performed   Instructor Signature

Name: _____

Collecting a clean-catch (midstream) urine specimen			
		yes	no
1.	Greets the patient. Identifies self by name and title.		
2.	Identifies the patient using 2 unique identifiers.		
3.	Explains the procedure to the patient.		
4.	Labels the specimen container in front of the patient, initialing and noting the time and date of collection. Asks the patient to confirm that the identifying information on the label is correct.		
5.	Correctly instructs the patient to collect the specimen.		
6.	Dons gloves.		
7.	Takes the urine specimen from the patient or retrieves it from the drop location.		
8.	Thanks the patient.		
9.	Places the specimen and the requisition or any required paperwork in the appropriate transport bag or container.		
10.	Removes gloves and washes hands.		

_____   _____
Date Reviewed   Instructor Signature

_____   _____
Date Performed   Instructor Signature

Name: _____

	Testing urine with reagent strips	yes	no
1.	Washes hands.		
2.	Puts on gloves.		
3.	Takes a strip from the bottle and recaps the bottle. Closes it tightly.		
4.	Dips the strip into the specimen.		
5.	Follows the manufacturer's instructions for when to remove the strip from the specimen. Removes the strip at the correct time.		
6.	Follows the manufacturer's instructions for how long to wait after removing the strip. After the proper time has passed, compares the strip with the color chart on the bottle. Does not touch the bottle with the strip.		
7.	Reads the results.		
8.	Stores the strips. Discards used items. Discards the specimen according to facility policy if further tests are not ordered.		
9.	Removes and discards gloves.		
10.	Washes hands.		
11.	Documents the procedure using facility guidelines.		

_____   _____
Date Reviewed   Instructor Signature

_____   _____
Date Performed   Instructor Signature

Name: _____

	Obtaining a throat culture	yes	no
1.	Greets the patient. Identifies self by name and title.		
2.	Identifies the patient using 2 unique identifiers.		
3.	Explains the procedure to the patient.		
4.	Gathers the required equipment.		
5.	Washes (or sanitizes) hands. Dons gloves and other PPE as required.		
6.	Removes the swab from its packaging.		
7.	Asks the patient to tilt head back slightly, open mouth, and say "Ahhhh."		
8.	Uses the tongue depressor to hold the tongue down and out of the way. Inserts the swab in the patient's mouth and rubs it along both of the patient's tonsils and the back of the throat, avoiding the uvula.		
9.	Removes the swab and tongue depressor and allows the patient to close his mouth.		
10.	Places the swab in its transport vial/tube. Breaks off the swab stick and/or breaks the culture medium ampule before sealing the tube if necessary.		
11.	Labels the tube in front of the patient, initialing and noting the time and date of the swab. Asks the patient (or parent/guardian) to confirm that the identifying information on the label is correct. Places the sealed tube and the requisition or any required paperwork in the appropriate transport bag or container. Properly discards any waste.		
12.	Thanks the patient (and parent/guardian, as appropriate).		
13.	Removes gloves and washes hands.		
14.	Documents the procedure according to facility policy.		

_____ _____
Date Reviewed   Instructor Signature

_____ _____
Date Performed   Instructor Signature

Name: _____

Practice Exam

Taking an Exam

Each agency offering certification for phlebotomy technicians has its own test format and rules. Exams from the most widely used and respected organizations generally have between 80 and 150 test questions with a time limit between 2 and 3 hours. Each certification agency has information on its website describing the exam. You should know how many questions you will have to answer and how much time you will have. Here are some general guidelines for taking exams to help you feel better prepared.

Your physical condition affects your mental abilities. Before taking an exam, get plenty of sleep and watch what you eat and drink. On the day of the exam, eat a healthy breakfast. It can be hard to think if you are hungry or if you did not eat a balanced breakfast. Avoid items such as soda and doughnuts, which contain simple sugars.

Being in good physical shape allows for more blood to get to the brain. If you get regular physical exercise, your body uses oxygen more effectively than it would if you were out of shape. Even exercising a few days before an exam can make a noticeable difference in thinking abilities.

When taking the exam, listen carefully to any instructions given. Be sure to read the directions and the questions carefully. If material seems unfamiliar, stay calm and reread the questions slowly. Try to eliminate answers for multiple choice questions that are clearly wrong. Your first choice is often correct, so do not change your answers unless you are sure of the correction.

Do not spend too much time on any one question. If you do not understand it, move on and go back if time and the test format allow. When you are finished with the test, review your answers if you can. Electronic tests vary in ability to go back to skipped questions and review answers before submission.

Remember that being nervous is natural. Most people get nervous before and during a test. A little stress can actually help you focus and make you more alert. Do not allow difficult questions to harm your confidence. Some questions will be challenging. Some may even cover material you have not learned or studied. This does not mean that you will not still pass the exam. Taking a few deep breaths may help you calm down. Remember that the work you have chosen to do is valuable and rewarding. Try to focus on this. The exam is your chance to show that you have learned how to perform this important job.

Note: There are 100 questions in this exam. The suggested time limit is 2 hours.

Practice Exam

1. If a phlebotomy technician receives a paper requisition with no tests marked they should
   (A) Look at the diagnosis code for guidance on what tests may be required
   (B) Draw an EDTA tube, a heparin tube, and a serum tube for a variety of specimens
   (C) Contact the provider for clarification
   (D) Ask the patient which tests were ordered

2. In addition to wearing gloves, what PPE should a phlebotomy technician wear when drawing blood from a patient who has an airborne illness?
   (A) A face shield
   (B) A gown
   (C) A surgical mask
   (D) An N95 respirator (or similar high-quality mask)

3. Which of the following should be done before a phlebotomy technician selects equipment for a blood draw?
   (A) Labels should be placed on tubes.
   (B) The patient should be greeted and properly identified.
   (C) The patient should be asked to sign a consent form for the blood draw.
   (D) The patient should tell the PBT which tests are ordered.

4. Which lancet size should be used for a capillary puncture on a 5-year-old child?
   (A) 0.85 mm
   (B) 1.5 mm
   (C) 2.2 mm
   (D) 2.5 mm

5. Which of these tubes contains an anticoagulant additive? (Choose 2.)
   (A) Tiger top
   (B) Red stopper
   (C) Green stopper
   (D) Orange stopper
   (E) Light blue stopper

6. What is the highest priority for a phlebotomy technician when a patient faints or has a seizure during a blood draw?
   (A) Preventing injury to the patient
   (B) Completing the draw
   (C) Preventing damage to laboratory equipment
   (D) Removing the tube that was filling

7. Which of the following is true of tearing the fingertip off of a glove before palpating a patient's arm?
   (A) It is a good way to improve the PBT's ability to find an appropriate site.
   (B) It should only be done if the PBT cannot feel the veins through the glove.
   (C) It contaminates the skin if the site has already been cleaned.
   (D) It should only be done if the PBT has lost track of which vein she was going to use.

8. A patient has orders for a CBC and a lipid panel. Which of these would be appropriate to draw?
   (A) 1 lavender tube
   (B) 1 red tube
   (C) 1 light blue tube and 1 green tube
   (D) 1 lavender tube and 1 tiger top tube

9. In the situation in question 8, which tube is drawn first?
   (A) Lavender
   (B) Tiger top
   (C) Light blue
   (D) Green

10. Which of the following is considered a unique identifier?
    (A) First name
    (B) Last name
    (C) Room number
    (D) Date of birth

11. Quality control checks on point-of-care devices are usually performed
    (A) Before each use
    (B) After each use
    (C) Daily
    (D) Weekly

12. A patient who has a phobia of needles refuses a blood draw. Which response by the phlebotomy technician is best?
    (A) "OK. I guess I can just tell your doctor she won't be able to find out what's wrong with you."
    (B) "I understand. Is there anything I could do to make this easier for you so we could get the tests your doctor ordered?"
    (C) "I get it. Needles terrify me, too."
    (D) "I'm afraid I can't let you leave without getting this draw done."

13. Which of these sets of equipment would be best for a 75-year-old cancer patient?
    (A) 18-gauge straight needle and evacuated tubes
    (B) 21-gauge straight needle and evacuated tubes
    (C) 23-gauge butterfly assembly and evacuated tubes
    (D) 23-gauge butterfly assembly and syringe with transfer device

14. A phlebotomy technician has selected a patient's basilic vein as a venipuncture site. When the needle is inserted the patient tells the PBT he feels a tingling sensation in his arm. What should the PBT do?
    (A) Remove the needle immediately
    (B) Tell the patient the procedure will be over quickly
    (C) Adjust the needle gently forward and backward to see if the sensation goes away
    (D) Tell the patient it is fine as long as there is no pain

15. Which of these tubes is a good choice for collecting a specimen for a CMP? (Choose 2.)
    (A) A gray-top tube
    (B) A green-top tube
    (C) A yellow-top tube
    (D) A lavender-top tube
    (E) A mottled-top (tiger top) tube

16. A phlebotomist working in a hospital is asked by a charge nurse to draw blood from the foot of a patient who has burns on her arms and hands. What should the PBT do?
    (A) Complete the draw
    (B) Ask the nurse for help with the draw
    (C) Ask the nurse if there is a written doctor's order for the draw
    (D) Ask the patient for confirmation and consent

17. Which of these situations can cause hemoconcentration?
    (A) The patient eating a fatty meal before a blood draw
    (B) The patient pumping their fist during site selection
    (C) The phlebotomist choosing a needle with a too-high gauge
    (D) The phlebotomist probing for a vein

18. A requisition notes that the patient's blood should be drawn 1 hour after he takes a dose of medication. The blood is likely being tested for
    (A) Peak medication levels
    (B) Trough medication levels
    (C) The presence of drugs of abuse
    (D) The medication's effect on red blood cell count

19. A hospital patient is having PT/INR tested daily. Yesterday PBT Jacob performed capillary puncture on the ring finger of the patient's right hand. Which of the following is a good possibility for today's puncture?
    (A) The pinky finger of the right hand
    (B) The ring finger of the right hand
    (C) The thumb of the right hand
    (D) The ring finger of the left hand

20. Which of these antiseptics contains alcohol and is generally not used when drawing blood for alcohol level testing?
    (A) Chlorhexidine gluconate
    (B) Povidone-iodine
    (C) Tincture of iodine
    (D) Antiseptic soap and water

21. PBT Angel is performing venipuncture on a patient who is obese. Which list best describes how he should approach this blood draw?
    (A) Ask the patient to let their arm dangle for 3–5 minutes before selecting a vein; consider using a blood pressure cuff as a tourniquet; ask the patient where blood draws have been successful in the past; use a longer needle
    (B) Ask the patient to pump their fist before selecting a vein; consider using a blood pressure cuff as a tourniquet; ask the patient where blood draws have been successful in the past; insert the needle at a 45-degree angle
    (C) Rub the patient's arm vigorously before selecting a vein; consider using a belt as a tourniquet; flick the patient's skin right before inserting the needle; use a longer needle
    (D) Ask the patient if they would mind having blood taken by finger stick rather than by venipuncture

22. If a PBT draws blood from 25 different patients in a day, how many pairs of gloves will the PBT use?
    (A) 1–8 pairs
    (B) 9–17 pairs
    (C) 18–24 pairs
    (D) 25 or more pairs

23. Filter paper is used to collect a _____ specimen for _____ testing.
    (A) Venipuncture, infant metabolic
    (B) Capillary, infant metabolic
    (C) Venipuncture, glucose
    (D) Capillary, glucose

24. Which of these lists the correct order of preference for venipuncture site selection?
    (A) Cephalic vein, basilic vein, median cubital vein
    (B) Median cubital vein, cephalic vein, basilic vein
    (C) Basilic vein, cephalic vein, median cubital vein
    (D) Median cubital vein, basilic vein, cephalic vein

25. Which of the following is a set of federal regulations regarding the staffing and operation of clinical laboratories?
    (A) CLIA
    (B) CLSI
    (C) CDC
    (D) HIPAA

26. What equipment should be used for venipuncture on a patient who is 43 years old, healthy, and has veins that appear to be of normal size and easy to locate?
    (A) An 18-gauge straight multisample needle and evacuated tubes
    (B) A 21-gauge straight multisample needle and evacuated tubes
    (C) A 21-gauge butterfly assembly and evacuated tubes
    (D) A 23-gauge butterfly assembly and a syringe/transfer device

27. A phlebotomy technician's supervisor reminds her to use a discard tube before drawing a light blue tube with a butterfly needle. Which of the following tubes is acceptable for use as a discard?
    (A) Green
    (B) Tiger
    (C) Light blue
    (D) Gray

28. Which of the following may be prevented by anchoring a patient's vein below the insertion site?
    (A) Blown vein
    (B) Rolling vein
    (C) Collapsed vein
    (D) Incomplete insertion into the vein

29. Which anticoagulant tube contains a reversible agent and allows laboratory technicians to perform clotting time tests on a specimen?
    (A) Oxalate tube
    (B) Heparin tube
    (C) EDTA tube
    (D) Citrate tube

30. A patient rolling up his sleeve and stretching out his arm is an example of
    (A) Express consent
    (B) Informed consent
    (C) Implied consent
    (D) Documented consent

31. How long can a tourniquet be left on a patient's arm before it must be removed?
    (A) 30 seconds
    (B) 60 seconds
    (C) 2 minutes
    (D) 5 minutes

32. Considering the collection tubes needed for each of these tests, which specimen would be drawn first?
    (A) Fasting blood glucose
    (B) D-dimer
    (C) C-reactive protein
    (D) Serum iron

33. Which of these patients should be called for a blood draw first?
    (A) A patient having peak medication levels tested who took the drug 30 minutes ago
    (B) A patient doing a glucose tolerance test who drank the glucose beverage 15 minutes ago
    (C) A patient whose requisition is marked *ASAP*
    (D) A patient who has not been fasting and whose requisition is marked *routine*

34. The volume of microcollection tubes is best measured in
    (A) Microliters
    (B) Liters
    (C) Cubic centimeters
    (D) Ounces

35. Using too small a venipuncture needle, pulling a syringe plunger back too forcefully, and "milking" the finger during capillary collection can all result in
    (A) Lipemic specimens
    (B) Icteric specimens
    (C) Hemoconcentrated specimens
    (D) Hemolyzed specimens

36. When a laboratory uses preprinted specimen labels, the phlebotomy technician
    (A) Will initial the tubes and mark them with the time and date after collection
    (B) Will initial the tubes and ask the patient to sign them after collection
    (C) Will initial the tubes and mark them with the patient's initials before calling the patient
    (D) Does not need to write anything on the tubes

37. In what situation might a point-of-care testing device not be disinfected after each use?
    (A) The device stays in a patient's room and is only used by that patient.
    (B) The device is only used on patients who have been confirmed to not have bloodborne illnesses.
    (C) The device is used on patients who share the same diagnosis.
    (D) The device is made of microbe-resistant material.

38. A pregnant patient with blood type A who is Rh-negative may have complications if she is carrying a fetus with which of these blood types?
    (A) O-
    (B) AB-
    (C) B-
    (D) A+

39. Which of these is an acceptable capillary puncture site for a newborn infant?
    (A) Arch of the foot
    (B) Big toe
    (C) Outside bottom of the heel
    (D) Third or fourth finger of either hand

40. A specimen that must be protected from light may be wrapped in _____ if an amber tube is not available.
    (A) Plastic wrap
    (B) Foil
    (C) Masking tape
    (D) A coin sleeve

41. After performing a fingerstick blood glucose test on a patient, a phlebotomy technician realizes it is past the expiration date printed on the test strip container. What should she do?
    (A) Repeat the test with an unexpired strip, taking blood from the same puncture site
    (B) Repeat the test with an unexpired strip, taking blood from a new puncture site on the same finger
    (C) Repeat the test with an unexpired strip, taking blood from a new puncture site on a different finger
    (D) Note in the LIS that the test was performed with an expired strip

42. What are 2 common vein formations in the antecubital fossa?
    (A) "A" and "B" formations
    (B) "H" and "M" formations
    (C) "X" and "Y" formations
    (D) "I" and "II" formations

43. Which tube is filled first during a capillary collection?
    (A) Nonadditive tube
    (B) Capillary blood gas tube
    (C) EDTA tube
    (D) Heparin tube

44. After how many unsuccessful attempts to draw blood should a phlebotomy technician ask for help from a supervisor?
    (A) 1
    (B) 2
    (C) 3
    (D) 4

45. Which of these choices describes one way in which blood culture collections are different from routine venipuncture collections?
    (A) The patient is placed in a supine position.
    (B) A nurse or other licensed professional must be present.
    (C) The venipuncture site is not cleaned as thoroughly.
    (D) The tops of the collection devices are cleaned.

46. When a tiger top tube is centrifuged, what are the resulting layers?
    (A) Clotted blood cells, separator gel, serum
    (B) Red blood cells, buffy coat, plasma
    (C) Clotted blood cells, buffy coat, serum
    (D) Red blood cells, separator gel, plasma

47. A phlebotomy technician who works as a substitute at different facilities arrives for a new assignment. The station where he is assigned to work has a standard phlebotomy chair, a bariatric chair, a stool for the phlebotomy technician, and a well-stocked supply cabinet between the chairs. There are biohazardous waste and standard trash cans close to the door. Across the room there is a counter with a sink, a centrifuge and other processing equipment, and a sharps receptacle. What should be changed?
    (A) The centrifuge should be in another area.
    (B) The 2 chairs should be immediately next to each other.
    (C) There is no need for a regular trash can.
    (D) The sharps receptacle should be within arm's reach of the phlebotomy chairs.

48. What happens first when a blood vessel is damaged?
    (A) Platelets are activated and begin plugging the wound.
    (B) A platelet and fibrin mesh is formed.
    (C) The blood vessel constricts.
    (D) An enzyme called *plasmin* is released.

49. Which of the following is the most common type of blood cell?
    (A) Lymphocytes
    (B) Erythrocytes
    (C) Granulocytes
    (D) Leukocytes

50. The Occupational Safety and Health Administration (OSHA) is a federal government agency that protects workers from
    (A) Hazards on the job
    (B) Lawsuits
    (C) Verbal abuse from residents
    (D) Unfair employment practices

51. When performing venipuncture, the PBT should insert the needle
    (A) Quickly and forcefully, bevel side up, at no lower than a 30-degree angle
    (B) Quickly and forcefully, bevel side down, at no lower than a 30-degree angle
    (C) In a single, fluid motion, bevel side up, at no higher than a 30-degree angle
    (D) In a single, fluid motion, bevel side down, at no higher than a 30-degree angle

52. What tests are commonly performed on stool? (Choose 2.)
    (A) Glucose
    (B) Occult blood
    (C) pH levels
    (D) Ova and parasites
    (E) *Helicobacter pylori*

53. Which of the following sends the most positive nonverbal message to a patient entering a drawing station?
    (A) The phlebotomy technician is looking down at specimen labels.
    (B) The phlebotomy technician glances up from gathering supplies.
    (C) The phlebotomy technician is looking intently at the patient.
    (D) The phlebotomy technician smiles and gestures to the phlebotomy chair.

54. A renal panel is a set of blood tests related to which body system?
    (A) The urinary system
    (B) The gastrointestinal system
    (C) The respiratory system
    (D) The nervous system

55. The additive in gray-topped tubes that prevents glycolysis is called
    (A) Acid citrate dextrose
    (B) Sodium fluoride
    (C) Sodium oxalate
    (D) Potassium oxalate

56. One reason that a phlebotomy needle should be inserted at as low an angle as possible is that this reduces the chance of striking
    (A) Muscle or bone
    (B) Bone or nerves
    (C) Nerves or arteries
    (D) Capillaries or arteries

57. What causes iatrogenic anemia?
    (A) A genetic defect
    (B) Blood loss due to conditions such as very heavy menstrual periods
    (C) Low iron levels
    (D) Excessive removal of a patient's blood

58. What supplies does a PBT need to make an ice slurry for specimen transport?
    (A) Cubed ice and a specimen bag
    (B) A commercial ice pack and a specimen bag
    (C) Crushed ice, water, and a specimen bag
    (D) Cubed ice, water, and a foam cooler

59. Which of the following is an adverse effect that can result from not properly identifying a patient or specimen?
    (A) The specimen is damaged and cannot be tested properly.
    (B) Diagnosis and treatment are delayed due to incorrect tests being performed.
    (C) The specimen is not prepared properly for testing.
    (D) The correct order of draw is not used.

60. What process occurs in capillary beds?
    (A) Blood is oxygenated.
    (B) Carbon dioxide is removed from the blood.
    (C) Exchanges of gases, nutrients, and wastes are made.
    (D) Blood is filtered.

61. A patient should be discouraged from bending their arm up after venipuncture because this may cause
    (A) The patient to pass out
    (B) The puncture wound to reopen
    (C) A hematoma
    (D) Hemolysis

62. A phlebotomy technician who often works in areas where radiation is used may have to wear
    (A) A dosimeter
    (B) Scrubs with a lead lining
    (C) A biohazard suit
    (D) Eye protection

63. A serum separator tube can be used when a patient has orders for
    (A) Complete blood count
    (B) Erythrocyte sedimentation rate
    (C) Coagulation testing
    (D) Comprehensive metabolic panel

64. A phlebotomist drew 2 tubes of blood from a patient and is preparing to label them. Which of the following describes the correct label placement?
    (A) One label should be placed lengthwise on each tube with the barcodes straight and unwrinkled.
    (B) One label should be placed horizontally so it can be wrapped around both tubes, holding them together.
    (C) One label should be placed horizontally on each tube in a spiral so that the barcodes are not covered.
    (D) One label should be placed horizontally on each tube with the ends stuck together like a tag.

65. Blood for donation is usually collected
    (A) By capillary puncture
    (B) With a syringe and transfer device
    (C) Using a 21-gauge needle
    (D) Using a 16-gauge needle

66. Which of the following is true about hand hygiene when a PBT's hands are not visibly soiled?
    (A) She does not need to perform hand hygiene.
    (B) She can use hand sanitizer.
    (C) She can rinse her hands rather than washing them with soap and water.
    (D) She can use friction for a shorter time while washing hands.

67. A person with type A+ blood
    (A) Has anti-A antibodies, B antigens, and has Rh factor on their red blood cells
    (B) Has anti-B antibodies, A antigens, and has Rh factor on their red blood cells
    (C) Has anti-A antibodies, B antigens, and does not have Rh factor on their red blood cells
    (D) Has anti-B antibodies, A antigens, and does not have Rh factor on their red blood cells

68. When would a phlebotomist see a *buffy coat* form in a blood specimen?
    (A) After a specimen without an anticoagulant additive has clotted
    (B) After a specimen with an anticoagulant additive has been chilled
    (C) After a specimen without an anticoagulant additive has been centrifuged
    (D) After a specimen with an anticoagulant additive has been centrifuged

69. Why should a PBT avoid performing capillary puncture on an edematous site?
    (A) It will be especially painful for the patient.
    (B) The skin will be difficult to penetrate with the lancet.
    (C) The blood will be diluted with excessive amounts of tissue fluid.
    (D) Platelet clumping will occur faster than it would at another site.

70. Blood that is dark red and must be drawn from the body is
    (A) Arterial blood
    (B) Venous blood
    (C) Capillary blood
    (D) Anticoagulated blood

71. The number associated with a requisition that can be used to trace specimens throughout the testing process is called a(n)
    (A) Accession number
    (B) Laboratory information number
    (C) Member record number
    (D) Authorization number

72. One reason venipuncture is rarely performed in the lower leg, ankle, or foot is because it may increase infection risk in patients with
    (A) Diabetes
    (B) High blood pressure
    (C) Arthritis
    (D) Alzheimer's disease

73. Which of the following is a safety rule related to centrifuge use?
    (A) Centrifuge anticoagulated tubes immediately if time allows.
    (B) Only operate the centrifuge with the load balanced.
    (C) Do not centrifuge specimens more than once.
    (D) Do not centrifuge specimens collected for whole blood testing.

74. According to CLSI patient identification standards, a patient should state and _____ her name and state her date of birth.
    (A) Write
    (B) Confirm
    (C) Spell
    (D) Click on

75. What is the most reliable method for finding a suitable vein for venipuncture?
    (A) Asking the patient
    (B) Visually inspecting the antecubital fossa
    (C) Looking in the patient's chart to see where blood was drawn previously
    (D) Palpation

76. Which of these tests is most likely to require chain of custody processes?
    (A) Pregnancy test
    (B) Glucose challenge test
    (C) Blood alcohol test
    (D) Type and crossmatch

77. What error may have been made by a phlebotomy technician if a specimen is marked *QNS*?
    (A) Left a tourniquet on too long
    (B) Did not allow a tube to fill completely
    (C) Did not mix additives properly
    (D) Used the wrong order of draw

78. One acceptable way to help a child who is frightened of a blood draw is to
    (A) Allow the child to watch another pediatric patient have blood drawn first
    (B) Ask the child to hold the gauze and bandage for you
    (C) Tell the child that much younger children have had their blood drawn and were not afraid
    (D) Tell the child they will get a reward for being brave

79. Which bloodborne illness is a serious risk to healthcare workers, but can be prevented with a vaccine that is provided at no cost by employers?
    (A) Hepatitis B
    (B) Hepatitis C
    (C) Human immunodeficiency virus
    (D) Tuberculosis

80. The Needlestick Safety and Prevention Act requires that employers involve employees in choosing
    (A) The type of soap used to clean accidental needlestick injuries
    (B) The location of sharps containers
    (C) The layout of phlebotomy stations
    (D) The safety devices on needles

81. Which of these follows the correct order of draw (venipuncture)?
    (A) Oxalate tube, heparin tube, serum tube
    (B) Serum tube, heparin tube, oxalate tube
    (C) Heparin tube, serum tube, oxalate tube
    (D) Serum tube, oxalate tube, heparin tube

82. After drawing a venipuncture specimen in a light blue-topped tube, what should a PBT do to ensure specimen quality?
    (A) Perform 8–10 inversions and be sure the tube is filled at least 50% to the fill line
    (B) Perform 8–10 inversions and be sure the tube is filled all the way to the fill line
    (C) Perform 3–5 inversions and be sure the tube is filled at least 50% to the fill line
    (D) Perform 3–5 inversions and be sure the tube is filled all the way to the fill line

83. What is the first thing a phlebotomy technician should do if he experiences an accidental needle stick?
    (A) Wash or flush the area immediately with soap and water for 20 seconds
    (B) Wash or flush the area immediately with soap and water for 15 minutes
    (C) Report the exposure to a supervisor
    (D) Report the exposure to the CDC

84. Aliquots are created by
    (A) Mixing together specimens from tubes with different additives
    (B) Mixing together specimens from tubes with the same additive
    (C) Dividing a specimen into smaller portions
    (D) Creating microscope slides from a specimen

85. What is the network of tissue that moves electrical signals through the heart?
    (A) The cardiac conduction system
    (B) The systemic circuit
    (C) The pulmonary circuit
    (D) The septum

86. At a minimum, how often do PBTs need to receive in-service training about bloodborne pathogens after their initial training?
    (A) Every month
    (B) Twice a year
    (C) Every year
    (D) Every 2 years

87. What are the 3 layers of the vein walls called?
    (A) The endocardium, epicardium, and pericardium
    (B) The tunica intima, tunica media, and tunica adventitia
    (C) The endotunica, epitunica, and peritunica
    (D) The proximal, medial, and distal layers

88. What is a common volume range for evacuated tubes used for pediatric patients?
    (A) 0.5–1.0 mL
    (B) 1.0–2.0 mL
    (C) 3.0–5.0 mL
    (D) 5.0–10.0 mL

89. Iodine-based antiseptics should not be used on patients who are allergic to
    (A) Gluten
    (B) Latex
    (C) Tree nuts
    (D) Shellfish

90. A syringe transfer device looks like a(n) _____ but is designed to attach securely to a syringe.
    (A) Evacuated tube holder
    (B) Butterfly assembly
    (C) Lancet
    (D) Collection tube

91. Why is the thumb not an acceptable site for capillary puncture?
    (A) Because it is often calloused
    (B) Because it is likely to be painful
    (C) Because there is a pulse point in the thumb and it is likely to bleed excessively
    (D) Because people use their thumbs often and it would interfere with daily activity

92. A phlebotomy technician has just completed a blood draw. She has thanked the patient and he has left. The specimens are placed in the proper location for processing. What should the PBT do now?
    (A) Check her schedule
    (B) Gather equipment for the next patient
    (C) Disinfect surfaces and wash hands
    (D) Call the next patient

93. What is the most common type of white blood cell?
    (A) Monocytes
    (B) Neutrophils
    (C) Lymphocytes
    (D) Eosinophils

94. Which of these actions is the best way for a phlebotomy technician to improve vein visibility?
    (A) Warming the site with a warm washcloth or commercial heating pack
    (B) Asking the patient to drink a glass of water
    (C) Asking the patient to jog in place or do other light exercise for 2 minutes
    (D) Rubbing the antecubital fossa briskly

95. How long should a PBT wait after removing a tourniquet before applying it to the same arm again?
    (A) It can be reapplied immediately.
    (B) After 30 seconds
    (C) After 1 minute
    (D) After 2 minutes

96. Performing venipuncture or capillary puncture on the same side of the body where a patient had a mastectomy increases the patient's risk for
    (A) Hematoma
    (B) Lymphoma
    (C) Lymphedema
    (D) Hemolysis

97. Which of the following is true of patients with phobias about needles and/or blood?
    (A) Their fears are irrational, so the PBT should proceed without addressing them.
    (B) It is usually best for the PBT to contact the patient's provider and arrange for some other kind of testing.
    (C) Their fears should not be dismissed, and the PBT should treat the patients with dignity.
    (D) With these patients it is best to perform the venipuncture when the patient is not expecting it.

98. Which antiseptic agent should be removed from a patient's skin with an alcohol prep pad after a procedure is complete?
    (A) Povidone-iodine
    (B) Tincture of iodine
    (C) Chlorhexidine gluconate
    (D) Antiseptic soap and water

99. Which of these tests may be performed on a specimen collected in a green-topped tube? (Choose 2.)
    (A) Calcium levels
    (B) Complete blood count
    (C) Cryoglobulins
    (D) D-dimer
    (E) Lipid panel

100. After _____ hours, fasting may affect certain analytes and make test results less accurate.
    (A) 8
    (B) 10
    (C) 12
    (D) 14

Name: _____

Name: _____

Name: _____